A Cross-Cultural Dialogue on Health Care Ethics

A Cross-Cultural Dialogue on Health Care Ethics

Edited by
Harold Coward and Pinit Ratanakul

Authors on the Research Team

Joan Anderson
Arthur Blue
Michael Burgess
Harold Coward
Robert Florida
Barry Glickman
Barry Hoffmaster
Edwin Hui
Edward Keyserlingk
Michael McDonald
Pinit Ratanakul
Sheryl Reimer Kirkham
Patricia Rodney
Rosalie Starzomski
Peter Stephenson
Khannika Suwonnakote
Sumana Tangkanasingh

Published for
The Centre for Studies in Religion & Society
by Wilfrid Laurier University Press

We acknowledge the financial support of the Government of Canada through the Book Publishing Industry Development Program for our publishing activities.

Canadian Cataloguing in Publication Data

A cross-cultural dialogue on health care ethics
Published for the Centre for Studies in Religion & Society.
Includes index.
ISBN 0-88920-325-3

1. Medical ethics. 2. Medical care – Cross-cultural studies. I. Coward, Harold G., 1936–. II. Ratanakul, Pinit.

R724.C76 1999   174′.2   C99-930548-4

© 1999
Wilfrid Laurier University Press
Waterloo, Ontario, Canada N2L 3C5

Cover design by Leslie Macredie

∞

Printed in Canada

A Cross-Cultural Dialogue on Health Care Ethics has been produced from camera-ready copy supplied by the Centre for Studies in Religion & Society.

Order from:
Wilfrid Laurier University Press
Waterloo, Ontario, Canada N2L 3C5

This book is dedicated to

our colleague

Attajinda Deepadung

who died before our work was completed

Table of Contents

Preface

This book is the result of the work of a Canada–Thailand interdisciplinary research team of the Centre for Studies in Religion and Society at the University of Victoria in Canada. The research team is interdisciplinary, composed of medical scientists, sociologists, anthropologists, psychologists, philosophers, and nursing, law, and religious studies scholars, split between Canada and Thailand. In Thailand, Mahidol University served as our research partner. In Canada, this project was co-sponsored by the Centre for Applied Ethics at the University of British Columbia, the Westminster Institute at the University of Western Ontario, and the Department of Native Studies, Brandon University. In terms of ethnic background, the research team included Caucasian, Aboriginal, Chinese, and Thai scholars. Community partners in Canada (all of whom serve a wide culture mix of clients) included: St Joseph's Hospital, Vancouver, B.C.; the Health Department, Vancouver, B.C.; the Open Arrow Clinic, Carberry, Manitoba; and the Inter-Community Health Centre of London, Ontario. The research work which spanned three years was funded by grants from the Social Sciences and Humanities Research Council of Canada and the Ford Foundation.

Special thanks are due to Centre staff June Bull and Ludgard De Decker for the support they provided the project. Ludgard De Decker saw the manuscript through the many steps required for publication. I also want to thank my colleagues Pinit Ratanakul, Michael McDonald, Joan Anderson, Barry Hoffmaster, Michael Burgess, and Patricia Rodney for their work in co-ordinating and editing various parts of the book.

This book is the result of the work of a large team encompassing many cultures, religions, and disciplines. To accomplish our research and writing, we had to learn to embody the kind of cross-cultural sensitivity and inter-cultural dialogue that we call for in health care ethics. This was not always easy, and was made possible only by the commitment and dedication to the project shown by all members of the research team. My thanks goes to each of them.

Harold Coward
Director
Centre for Studies in Religion and Society
University of Victoria
Victoria, B.C.

Chapter 1
Introduction

Harold Coward and Pinit Ratanakul

The ethical theories employed in health care today assume, in the main, a modern Western philosophical framework which is then applied to issues such as abortion, euthanasia, consent, and organ transplantation. The application of this approach to non-Western and traditional cultures needs critical examination. The diversity of cultural and religious assumptions regarding human nature, health and illness, life and death, and the status of the individual suggested to us that a cross-cultural study of health care ethics is needed. This is especially evident in the engagement of modern Western biomedical ethics with Asian cultures and Aboriginal traditions. On the one hand, there is the multicultural context in which health care operates in Canadian and American cities – think of Vancouver, Toronto, Montreal, Chicago, or San Francisco. On the other, there is the export of modern Western biomedicine (with its European scientific worldview) to other cultures (with their very different worldviews) in a colonizing fashion – "colonizing" because aspiring young people from Thailand, China, India, or Aboriginal cultures are brought to medical schools or ethics departments in

European or North American universities, trained in modern biomedicine or ethics, with little or no reference to their own cultures and traditional medicines, and sent home to establish and practise modern biomedicine and its associated ethics in their home cultures. Often this has been done in an insensitive and imperialistic fashion – hence the use of the term "colonizing". Sometimes, however, both in distant home cultures and in the multicultural contexts of North American cities, the interaction of modern and traditional medicine (and their very different worldviews) has occurred with a sensitivity that is not at all imperialistic or one-sided but betrays an understanding of the complementary strengths each approach has to offer. Members of our research team, both individually and as a group, have learned from such experiences. Let us consider a couple of examples.

Our research team was composed of mixed backgrounds: Christian, secular, Aboriginal, Chinese – faculty members all from medicine, nursing, biology, anthropology, philosophy, law, or religion – and Thai Buddhists (also faculty members from philosophy, nursing, and sociology). Our team meetings were held in both Canada and Thailand. During a visit to Thailand we made a field trip to a village about 90 kilometres outside Bangkok. There we found two medical units serving the community: a modern biomedical clinic and a monk-healer practising in the nearby Buddhist Temple. The monk-healer specialized in treating simple fractures without casts or splints but with daily hot herbal oil massage and Buddhist chanting. The patients slept in the Temple on simple cots and ate food provided by their families. The Temple and the monk-healer depended on freewill offerings from the village and treated patients free of charge. The cure of the fractured limbs was very rapid and successful, partly because the leg or arm was not immobilized. Recognition of this was given by the nearby biomedical clinic which referred simple fracture cases to the monk-healer for treatment. In their view, his treatment was better and certainly more cost-effective than they could offer. The monk-healer, however, recognized that his technique was not suitable for compound fractures, which he referred to the biomedical clinic for treatment. In this way, the wisdom and skills of both cultures – modern Western biomedicine and traditional Buddhist monk-healers – with their very different worldviews and approaches, functioned together in a co-operative and complementary way. To us this seemed a good example of what can happen when modern Western biomedicine sees itself to be one cultural approach to health care alongside others. In such a context, ethical questions can be resolved by examining the ethical principles present in each culture, critically assessing each other's values, and identifying common values found within all traditions.

This example points up the most fundamental finding of our research. In response to our initial question, "How does one train doctors, nurses, social workers, chaplains, medical ethicists, pharmacists, and hospital administrators to be sensitive to other cultures?", our research led us to a surprising conclusion – namely, that modern Western biomedicine and its health care system is itself a culture with its own belief system, social structure, initiation rituals, language, dress, and educational system. Modern Western medicine does not occupy a neutral position from which to relate itself sensitively to other cultures. Rather modern Western medicine is itself a culture alongside the other cultures – Muslim, Buddhist, Hindu, Chinese, etc. Even for those of us who come from a Christian background and have grown up in Canada or the United States, entry into the hospital for surgery or treatment is an experience of entering another world which seems quite foreign to us. As we go through Admitting, we feel ourselves to be entering a world which operates by its own rules over which we have little control. If we want treatment, we must trust and submit ourselves to this new medical culture. Only those who have had medical training or previous patient experience understand what is happening – because they have been cultured into the biomedical worldview.

Is this what happens when we visit the biomedical culture? Sometimes, with a sensitive and open doctor, nurse, clinic or hospital, it is. However, the experience may be an imperialistic and insensitive superimposition of the biomedical culture upon you. You are taken from family and friends and placed in unfamiliar surroundings filled with strange sights, smells, sounds, and food – to say nothing of the technology to which one is asked to submit. Modern biomedical culture operates with its own norms and standards covering everything from architectural design, forms of consent, and standards of purity. Nothing is wrong with this biomedical culture in and of itself, so long as it does not make itself God – sees itself as embodying the absolute truth (modern medical science) to which all other cultures must unquestioningly submit. Modern Western biomedicine has much wisdom to offer humankind, as do most cultures. But as with our experience of other cultures, we find shortcomings, along with points of new value. The same should be true of our experience of the modern biomedical culture. Ethical sensitivity requires that modern Western biomedicine, whether practised in a Canadian clinic or a Thai hospital, recognize itself to be a distinctive culture and interact with other cultures in a sensitive and respectful rather than imperialistic way.

While in Thailand, our research team also encountered examples of the colonial and imperialistic export of modern biomedicine. Unlike their country cousins, hospital staff in Bangkok viewed the biomedicine that they had learned in the West as absolute scientific truth. They gave no recognition to the traditional medicine of the monk-healers. We might say that they were "new converts" to modern Western biomedicine. As a result, in Bangkok, unlike the village we visited, hospitals and clinics would not work in co-operation with the monk-healers. Patients who went to both were afraid to tell the doctors or nurses for fear of being reprimanded or refused treatment. Even though most of the medical staff were Buddhist, their Western training had led them to privilege biomedicine and its Western worldview and ethics over their own Buddhist culture, values, and traditional medicine. This has also led to unethical decision making with regard to government financial allocations to support Health Care in Thailand. The majority of Thailand's health care budget is allocated to the hospitals and clinics practising biomedicine. Very little support is given to the monk-healers, who carry a heavy burden in providing health care for those in need. In one area, however, the monk-healers are recognized. The city hospitals and clinics do refer terminal cases to the monk-healers for palliative care. This the monk-healers provide in a most compassionate fashion, without turning anyone away, yet without government support. In this way the state is spared considerable expense, while the growing need for care of the terminally ill is unfairly downloaded on the monks.

Canada has not escaped policy problems in the area of the interaction between modern and traditional medicine. In Vancouver, for example, there is a large Chinese population and traditional Chinese herbal medicine is popular and widely practised. At the same time, many Chinese people go to the doctor for modern medicine. Both the doctor and the Chinese herbalist end up prescribing for the same ailment in ignorance of each other. Since herbal prescriptions also contain potent drugs, the patient is in danger of taking two forms of drugs from two separate medicines that could produce a tragic result.

Doctors and nurses who have studied Chinese herbal medicine have become aware of this danger. How to solve the problem? An immediate response is that since the Chinese herbal remedies contain powerful substances, they should be regulated by Canada's Food and Drug Act. Indeed, such legislation has been proposed by the Government of Canada and only recently withdrawn for further review. While at first blush this proposal seems reasonable, we need to consider the cultural implications of such a policy approach. It could well mean that Chinese herbs, as controlled drugs, would be taken over by the pharmaceutical companies and only be available from Western-style pharmacists in drug stores. This would put the traditional Chinese herbalist out of business and result in the loss of one form of traditional Chinese medicine. Our well-intentioned worry over the potentially dangerous double prescription of drugs for a Chinese patient will have led to a policy solution in which the traditions of biomedicine are superimposed upon Chinese herbal medicine in such a way as to effectively kill it. By the way, the same danger is present in our engagement with the herbalists in Aboriginal cultures. Rather than learning from them and working with them in culturally sensitive ways, our concern for regulative public policy can easily have the unintended result that this last aspect of Aboriginal culture is being taken over by the white-man – namely the pharmaceutical industry which is part and parcel of modern biomedicine.

Do not misunderstand us. We are not saying that all public policy decisions produce destructive results in cross-cultural situations. We *are saying* that there is a real danger when the power and dominance of modern biomedicine over the cultural/religious herbal traditions is as strong as it is in many countries today. To avoid a destructive imperialistic result, we will have to make health care policy which deals with dangers to the public – but does it in ways that are culturally sensitive and do not result in the destruction of alternative traditional medicines. Our analysis of ethics in regard to health care policy is offered in Part IV of this book.

Part I begins with a critical examination of the concepts of culture, health, and illness from a cross-cultural perspective. In addition to modern bio-medicine learning to recognize itself as a separate culture, our analysis in Part I points out that as a child of European Enlightenment thought, biomedicine assumes that the identity of a person is as an individual rather than as a part of a group. This has important ethical implications – such as who gives consent, the individual or the group? Those of us who have grown up in the modern West are often insensitive to the deep cultural and religious issues involved. Let us illustrate with an incident from Harold Coward's experience. He writes as follows:

Many years ago when I was just beginning my career as a university professor, I ended up going to a conference with a colleague who was Hindu, born in India. Now I knew all about Hinduism – in fact I taught it in the university. But until this trip I had not really understood the tradition from within. The difference began when we selected our seats on the plane. Of course, we would sit together, but the seats should be chosen so as to avoid certain inauspicious numbers. When we got to the hotel room which we were sharing, other things began to happen. I noticed my friend using my toothpaste. For me, this seemed to be an invasion of my privacy and property, without even the courtesy of asking permission. For him, there was no clear separation of ownership because we were together – our identities and possessions were merged into a collective unity. It was our toothpaste, and as it looked interesting, he was trying it. I soon came to understand that being together also meant that whenever we left the room to attend sessions, eat, or do some sightseeing, we did it together. This was quite different from my usual conference-going experience of room sharing where the only time you might see your roommate was at night or on waking in the morning. Being with my Hindu colleague and sharing his worldview meant we did everything together. The two of us were merged into one. For me to go off to do something on my own would have caused a serious rupture in our collective personhood. No longer was I an autonomous individual. We made our decisions as a shared identity.

The collective as opposed to individual identity, illustrated in Coward's narrative, has important implications for issues of diagnosis, treatment, and consent. As doctors, nurses, social workers, ministers, or ethicists, it means we may not interact with an autonomous person (our usual experience), but with a person who understands their self-identity in terms of a larger whole, such as an extended family.

Alan Roland, a New York psychiatrist, reports just such an experience (Roland 1988). He found that his Indian Hindu patients (highly educated professionals) did not respond to his usual modern Western therapies, which assumed a strongly individualized sense of self – an I-ness characterized by a self-contained set of ego boundaries with sharp distinctions between self and others. Instead he found his South Asian patients to be a familial or "we-self" that enabled them to function within extended families. Rather than the self-contained ego boundaries of the typical North American "I-self" which allows us to function in a highly autonomous society, the "we-self" of his Indian patients had highly permeable ego boundaries opening the way for the constant empathy and receptivity to others necessary for life in an extended family. Instead of actualization of the individual self, the personal and spiritual goal of the South Asian is the reciprocal responsibility required to live in harmony within the hierarchical structure of family, society, and ideally all of nature. Whereas the North American "I-self" sharply separates between self and others, self and nature, often in a competitive fashion, the "we-self" of Eastern cultures extends outward to include family, caste-group, linguistic–ethnic culture and even the natural environment. From the Buddhist perspective, which is dominant in the cultures of East and South-east Asia, it is our false attachment to the "I-self" and its selfish desires that is the cause of unethical action and of suffering. Understanding ourselves as but a tiny interdependent part of the complex "we-self" of the cosmos leads to compassionate action and *Nirvana*. Yet within that complex "we-self", observes Roland, a highly private ego is maintained.

What does all this mean for health care? First, diagnosis and treatment in many cultures will have to pay more attention to the extended family and the environmental context in which the person lives – the "we-self". For example, says Coward,

> my wife, a nurse, working in a family practice unit serving Aboriginal patients had frequent "we-self" experiences. When a young woman would arrive with gynecological problems, she would be accompanied by her mother, aunts, and grandmother. All would insist on going back to the

examining room together (a room designed to hold just two or three). When the doctor was taking the history, it would be the grandmother who would do all the talking, saying when the girl had had her last period, etc. Everyone knew everything, naturally, as they were a "we-self". And everyone expected to be involved in the treatment and any ethical decisions to be made.

This raises the second point, namely that issues of consent have to take seriously that the ethical decision maker in such a culture is not just the individual but the "we-self" of which they are but a part. Recognition of this fact should cause us to re-examine our methods and forms for obtaining consent, which, for the most part, are devised on the assumption that the person is an autonomous individual – an "I-self", sharply separated from others in one's family or society. The existence of cultures with "we-self" expanding identities challenges autonomous conceptions of health and human rights often assumed in UN declarations, especially relating to women and children. We should not be surprised to discover that the feminist movements in traditional cultures do not always express the goal for women in terms of individual women's rights. Rather it is the just and respected place of women within the "we-self" of the family that is the focus of ethical analysis. When ethical issues surrounding reproduction arise, a woman within the "we-self" ponders the good of the extended family, along with her own desires, in coming to a decision. Nor should we be surprised to find that in such cultures the idea that children or adolescents have ethical standing independent of the family raises reactions of incomprehension and hostility.

While our modern Western notions of individual autonomy and human rights can serve to highlight ethical abuses and exploitation that can and do arise in the extended family, the other side of the coin is that the "we-self" ideals of mutual responsibility and respect between ourselves, others, and the environment are a much needed corrective to a self-centred selfishness that our North American competitive "I-self" so successfully generates. Indeed at a time of tightened resources in health care, ethical questions of who gets treatment and in what order of priority are made very difficult, if not impossible to resolve, when the rights of individual autonomy reign supreme. We are also led, even in our quest for health, to exploit the environment in unsustainable ways. The new field of environmental health is leading us to see that it is both unethical and ineffective to think of our health as individual persons separate from our concern for all of nature, of which we are but a part. If our pharmaceutical and health care industries, along with the cities we live in, are not in a sustainable relationship with nature, our efforts to achieve health may be for naught. As Aboriginal and Buddhist wisdom teaches, our cross-cultural sensitivity must extend out not only to other human cultures but ultimately to the animals, plants, earth, air, and water – if we are to achieve good health. Seeing ourselves as individuals (I-selves) separate from other humans and from nature fosters an ethic of self-interest rather than an ethic of identification with the larger whole – humanity or the cosmos. It produces a focus on human rights (often defined as isolated individual rights in health care law and policy) as a way of ensuring that each person gets his or her fair share of the health care resources. It fosters a health care economy, which when meshed with modern technology, constantly expands to supply ever enlarging needs and an expanding world population. The result can easily become an unsustainable degradation of nature in the name of serving human health needs, defined as human rights. Human beings and their needs are put at war with the sustainability of nature – which, according to some readings of Bible and Qur'an, is created for the purpose of supporting humans. This one-sided ontology may have helped foster the modern liberal emphasis on the individual. But when put together with utilitarian secular ethics and the market economy, the results for the global ecosystem and for human health may be devastating.

A collective "we-self" sense of personhood, by contrast, may provide a more practical and helpful ethical approach, one which strives to balance the needs of the individual with those of the larger interdependent whole. In our current and future scarce resources scenarios, we may find wisdom in the way traditional "we-self" cultures have developed ethical guidelines for solving such problems. Not only ought we consider the health care needs of others, in other cultures and other parts of the world, but, says Aboriginal ethics, we must leave enough for seven generations into the future. In traditional Islamic, Hindu, Buddhist, and Chinese societies self-identity is constructed not by individual choices (as tends to be our modern way) but by participating in a "family" which may extend out to include caste, tribe, and all humans as well as plants, animals, and the cosmos. For example, in the Chinese worldview, it is never the isolated, individual "self" but the "self" as interrelated in community, nature, and with heaven that is the ethical agent. Identity and health are one's harmonious interrelationships, not in one's choices/rights, powers, and privileges. Such a broadened understanding of self and health leads to a focus on obligations to the whole rather than an emphasis on individual human rights – although the safeguards of the latter are an important defence against abuses of the individual (especially the poor, children, and women) that the former has sometimes produced, and therefore they need to be retained but balanced. Such a need to produce a better balance between individual rights and social responsibilities, between the self and relationship, is now being recognized in the work of some contemporary philosophers and religious thinkers in the West – a move toward "communitarianism". The values and worldviews of Eastern peoples can be of help in analysing the bases for such a balance.

Ethical issues such as those illustrated above are given detailed analysis in Part I. In chapter 2, Pinit Ratanakul takes us into the Thai Buddhist worldview and its quite different perceptions of health and disease. And in chapter 3, Hui introduces us to the concepts of health and disease in Traditional Chinese Medicine which functions in an equal and complementary fashion with biomedicine in the Republic of China. Anderson and Kirkham (chapter 4) point out that there are no universal norms of health. Conceptions of health and illness vary across individuals and cultures, embodying spiritual and social as well as physical factors. For example, a person may report feeling healthy even in the face of impending death from cancer. While the World Health Organisation definition of health adds social and environmental factors, a feminist and post-colonial analysis exposes the systematic injustice for the poor, the coloured, and women, incorporated into many conceptions of health. Health and illness, they show, must be viewed holistically as including relationships with food, family, and nature. Ethical issues go beyond the just allocation of resources within health care and raise issues of social justice for social groups that have been marginalized or oppressed – with these factors being the key determinants of health for them. Stephenson (chapter 5) examines expanding notions of culture including seeing medicine as itself a culture rather than a neutral scientific truth. He also explores the way cultural collectives are threatened by the ascendant individualism which often dominates modern medicine. To close out the conceptual considerations of Part I, McDonald (chapter 6) asks "can we have a shared normative basis for health care ethics that is sensitive to cultural and religious differences?" Christopher Boorse's proposal that health and health care are value-free is examined alongside various evaluative conceptions of health.

In Part II, we offer some selected examples of how these different conceptions of health and health care ethics manifest themselves – especially in beginning- and end-of-life situations. Brief presentations of the Buddhist, Chinese, Christian, and modern secular views are offered to introduce the reader to a range of cultural/religious perspectives and the differences they make for ethics in birth and death considerations.

Ethical issues in the delivery of health care ethics are discussed in Part III. Chapter 10 focuses on parental refusal of life-saving treatment for children. The case of K'aila, a baby born to Aboriginal parents in Alberta, is featured. Two types of knowledge and authority are opposed: the physician (modern biomedicine) and the parents (Aboriginal). In K'aila's case the physician determined that a liver transplant was the only means of preserving the baby's life. The parents, however, refused on the basis of their cultural and religious beliefs that a transplanted organ from another person would bring that person's spirit into their child thus impoverishing K'aila by recreating him, not as himself but as someone else. According to current law in Canada, parents' authority in such a case can be overridden if they are thought to be not acting in the best interests of the child. The physician argued that the transplant should go ahead so that the child could live until old enough to make up his own mind about adopting his parent's religious and cultural views. Here the physician is assuming that his own view of the person as an autonomous individual, composed mainly of a physical body, should dominate. By contrast the parents had a different notion of what it was about K'aila that they had a responsibility to protect and nurture – his spirit rather than his physical body. The chapter goes on to explore how the case of K'aila would be dealt with in a Thai Buddhist or a Hindu culture. Chapter 11 offers a counterpoint to the K'aila case study of the previous chapter. In a comparison of notions of autonomy, informed consent, and personal choice in contemporary Euro-North American and Aboriginal North American patients, Keyserlingk finds much in common. Both patient groups, he argues, share in a belief that there may be metaphysical causes of illness and make decisions not as individuals but with their families. In his view it is not so much the cultural variable that is crucial but rather the degree of sensitivity exhibited by the physician and the health care givers. Finally in this section on the delivery of health care ethics, chapter 12 examines ethical decisions surrounding death. Autonomy approaches typical of the modern West are compared with Canadian Hutterite and Thai Buddhist approaches in which the social and spiritual significance of death and dying dominate.

Part IV of the book brings the ethical considerations of our cross-cultural dialogue to bear on health policy issues. Chapter 13 offers a critical assessment of North American health care policy. Legal recourse is increasingly made necessary by the impersonal cultural context in which much health care is delivered. And there are systemic inequities having to do with geography (urban versus rural), gender (women often have less opportunity and are in more need), and public participation (the majority dominates at the expense of minorities). In chapter 14, threats to traditional medicines in Canada (Chinese herbology) and Thailand (monk-healers) by the biomedical paradigm are examined. Finally, chapter 15 offers some ethical observations surrounding the use of medicinal plants, food supplements, and vitamins. The interest of the pharmaceutical industry in what Glickman calls "green medicines" is assessed.

This book does not attempt to be comprehensive. Rather it aims at exemplifying the dialogue between cultures (of which modern biomedicine is one) which is needed if the ethics of health care is to develop a global awareness and sensitivity to and respect for the diversity of peoples and their values. It is to be hoped that such dialogue will not only advance understanding but will help to foster a greater balance and a fuller truth in consideration of the human condition and what makes for health and wholeness in its members.

Reference

Roland, Alan. 1988. *In search of self in India and Japan: Toward a cross-cultural psychology*. Princeton: Princeton University Press.

Part I

Culture, Health, and Illness

Part I, Introduction

Michael McDonald

Many writers in each section of this book take multiple perspectives on cross-cultural health care issues. These perspectives have been shaped and enriched by a process of dialogue that extended over three years. While cross-cultural dialogue is not an easy process, it can be a rewarding one. We are thus a diverse group involved in a dialogue about diversity itself.

Part I is a discussion about a multiplicity of problems that confront society, health care professionals, and clients. Key concepts such as culture, religion, health, and illness are often contested in plural societies comprised of many different kinds of people. Even when they are not contested and taken for granted, understanding the assumptions that lie behind them can be crucial for dealing with major ethical issues in health care. For example, health may well be defined and understood as a positive state of being in societies, while in others illness is the defining category and health becomes a residual concept defined in a negative way as people who are not sick. The meanings of health and illness are often constructed in religious and philo-sophical terms, and the treatment of people predicated on existential terms that are the essence of cultural configurations of living. We recognize that cultures are expressed in beliefs and practices. In our work, we try to explore the assumptions that lie behind these beliefs and practices, recognizing that we must begin by trying to unmask our own assumptions. We are acutely aware that our interpretations of other people's belief systems and practices are refracted through the lenses of our own systems of meaning.

Belief systems and practices can be explored along a variety of axes: theological, economic, philosophical, political, legal, and so forth. These explorations can also be conducted in a variety of ways using the diverse methodologies and tools of different disciplines. All of these are important for understanding the quality of interpersonal connections that are at the core of ethical decision making.

In Part I, we examine different ways of talking about culture, health, and illness, which themselves reflect values and choices, not only within the "Western" or modern context but also in the Chinese and Thai contexts. In doing this, we recognize that how we construct these central but contested concepts has implications not only for the practice of health care, but also for various discourses on health care ethics and how issues of social justice are ultimately addressed. Without essentializing the notion of health as a good with a single meaning for all people at all times and places, we believe that a powerful case can be made for a decent minimum of the material conditions that contribute to health and well-being. This has profound implications for the provision and distribution not only of the various elements of health care, but also for those factors like wealth and power that have such a profound impact on health status.

In his chapter, Pinit Ratanakul weaves together the Buddhist account of health and disease and delivery of health care in both traditional and modern forms in Thailand. In his chapter, Edwin Hui takes a similar perspective by first examining the concepts of health and disease in Traditional Chinese Medicine and then considering actual processes of health delivery in contemporary China. Anderson and Reimer Kirkham, in their critical perspective on discourses on health, examine negative and positive concepts of health and the ways in which the theoretical and practical uses of these concepts often reflect unequal social relationships, based on race, gender, and class. Peter Stephenson then discusses and deconstructs various understandings of culture particularly as they are embodied in Western health care and medical ethics. These are explored through a series of examples in which culture appears in various guises, some universalistic in their claims and others particularistic. Finally, in Michael McDonald's examination of health and culture, there is a discussion of whether the recognition of the diversity of perspectives on health and illness undermines the possibility of cross-cultural agreement on major social choices with respect to health care.

Chapter 2
Buddhism, Health, Disease, and Thai Culture

Pinit Ratanakul

Therevada Buddhism, also known as the Hinayana tradition, has been considered the core of Thai national identity since the establishment of the first Kingdom of Sukhodhaya in the thirteenth century. Though the present constitution does not make it compulsory for every Thai to follow the Buddhist beliefs and practices, it requires the king to be a Buddhist. For the vast majority of the Thai population one cannot be a true Thai without being a Buddhist. Since early times the Thai *sangha*, the order of Buddhist monks, has been integrated into the state structure to provide legitimation for the monarch and/or political rulers. The institution of kingship, Buddhism, and nation are considered as the basic triad of social solidarity and identity. They have been so intermingled in the course of history and are so deeply meaningful to the hearts of the people as to form the dominant core of Thai culture. In this culture, although one may notice the elements of Brahmanism and animism in the belief and customs of Thai people, Buddhism remains the basis in the moulding and development of Thai cultural values. And one cannot understand or appreciate Thai culture without having some basic comprehension of Buddhist tenets. With its holistic worldview, its principle of "dependent origination", and its ideal of compassion, Buddhism has undergirded the Thai cultural understanding of health and approach to health care.

Buddhist worldview and dependent origination

The Buddhist holistic worldview is primarily based on a belief in the interdependence of all phenomena and a correlation between mutually conditioning causes and effects. This belief is formulated by the principle of dependent origination, also referred to as the law of conditionality, the causal nexus that operates in all phenomena – physical, psychological, and moral. In the physical realm, for example, all things in the universe are intimately interrelated as causes and effects without beginning and end. And the world is an organically structured world where all of its parts are interdependent. Similarly in human society every component is interrelated. The same is also found in the psycho-physical sphere, in which the mind and the body are not separate units but an interdependent part of the overall human system.

The Buddhist worldview also comprises a belief in *kamma*, the correlation between deed and its subsequent consequences, as in the moral realm this principle of dependent origination operates by the name of the law of *kamma* stating the conditionality of this causal relation.[1] This implies that the Buddhist law of *kamma* does not entail complete determinism. If such a determinism were accepted there would be no possibility of the eradication of suffering. A man would ever be bad for it is his *kamma* to be bad. But this is not so and the effect of *kamma* can be mitigated not only in one life but even beyond, as according to Buddhism life is not limited to a single, individual existence. Present life is only a part of the round of existence (*samsara*) which stretches out across space and time. A single existence is conditioned by others proceeding it and in turn conditions one or a series of successive existences. Existence is thus at the same time an effect in one respect and a cause in another. This imprisonment in the round of existence is the result of one's own deeds (*kamma*), good or bad. Conditioned by deeds, the present form of existence can be changed or dissolved by deeds. This is possible because the present is not the *total* effect of the past. It is simultaneously cause and effect. As an *effect*, we are conditioned by the causal matrix made up of the social and biological continuities of life themselves and thus are the effect of our past deed. What we are now is the result of what we have been before. But as a *cause*, we are the absolute master of our destiny. The present, though elusive, is the building block of the future. What we shall be depends on what we are and shall do, with our own choice.

Dependent origination, health, and kamma

Within this worldview, health and disease involve the overall state of a human being and are interwoven with many factors such as economics, education, social and cultural milieu. All these conditional factors need to be seriously taken into account in the understanding of health and disease. Health is therefore to be understood in terms of holism. It is the expression of harmony – within oneself, in one's social relationships, and in relation to the natural environment. To be concerned about a person's health means to be concerned with the whole person, his (her) physical and mental dimensions, social, familial, and work relationships, as well as the environment in which he (she) lives and which acts on him (her). Therefore the tendency to understand health only in relation to particular parts of the human organism such as the defects is unacceptable to Buddhism. In the Buddhist holistic perspective, disease is the expression of the disturbed harmony in our life as a whole. By its physical symptoms, disease draws our attention to this disturbed harmony. Hence healing in Buddhism is not the mere treatment of these measurable symptoms. It is more an expression of the combined effort of the mind and the body to overcome disease than a fight between medicine and disease. Its real aim is to enable the patient to bring back harmony within himself and in his relationships with the others and the natural environment. In this context healing is not an end in itself, but rather a means by which medicine helps to serve the value of human health and well-being.

Apart from this holistic approach, Buddhism attributes *kamma* as an important contributing factor to health and disease. In the Buddhist perspective good health is the correlated effect of good *kamma* in the past and vice versa. This interpretation of health and disease in terms of *kamma* is to emphasize that there is a relationship between morality and health. Health depends on our life-styles, i.e. the way we think, the way we feel, and the way we live. Illness is the consequence of an unhealthy life-style such as one characterized by sensual indulgence, for example. This is the normativistic component of the Buddhist perspective on health which involves the practice of moral and religious values such as compassion, tolerance, and forgiveness. This is the underlying reason why Buddhism advises those who want to be healthy to practise morality (*sila*), mental discipline (*samadhi*), and wisdom (*panna*), in the Noble Eightfold Path.

Perhaps we will understand the role of *kamma* in health and illness as we look at the following cases. For example, in the time of an epidemic there are usually some people who succumb while others escape even though both groups are exposed to the same conditions. According to the Buddhist view the difference between the former and latter is due to the nature of *kamma* of each in the past. Other examples are the cases where though the treatment given was successful the patient died, and where in spite of ineffective treatment the patient lived. There have also been cases of remarkable and unexpected recoveries when modern medicine has given up all hope for remission. Such cases strengthen the Buddhist belief that besides the physical cause of disease, illness can be the effect of bad *kamma* in past lives. A disease with a kammic cause cannot be cured until that kammic result is exhausted. But the *kamma* of every person is a mystery both to himself and others. Hence no ordinary person can definitely know which disease is caused by *kamma*. Therefore one has to be careful in imputing *kamma* especially for disease because it may lead to a fatalistic attitude of not seeking any cure at all or giving up treatment out of despair. Buddhism advises us that for practical purposes we have to look upon all diseases as though they are produced by mere physical causes. And even if the disease has a *kammic* cause it should be treated. As no condition is permanent and as the causal relation between deed and its correlated consequence is more conditional than deterministic there is the possibility for the disease to be cured so long as life continues. On the other hand we cannot tell at what point the effect of bad *kamma* will be exhausted. Therefore we need to take advantage of whatever means of curing and treatment are available. Such treatment, even if it cannot produce a cure, is still useful because appropriate physical and psychological conditions are needed for the kammic effect to take place. The presence of a predisposition to certain diseases through past *kamma* and the physical condition to produce the disease will provide the opportunity for the disease to arise. But having a certain treatment will prevent a bad kammic result manifesting fully. This kind of treatment does not interfere with the working of the individual *kamma* but reduces its severity. The advice of Buddhism to a person with an incurable disease is to be patient and to perform good deeds to mitigate the effects of the past bad *kamma*. At least the individual effort to maintain or recover is itself good *kamma*.

The belief in *kamma* in relation to health and disease does not lead to fatalism, nor to pessimism. As mentioned before, the law of *kamma* does not rule with an iron hand or bring a curse. This law only stresses the causal relation between cause and effect. It does not entail complete determinism. To believe in *kamma* is to take personal responsibility for health. Health is not given. It has to be gained by one's own efforts, and one should not blame others for the suffering one is going through because of the disease. Besides, it may be a comfort to think that our illness is no fault of our present lives but the legacy of a far distant past, and that by our own attitudes and efforts towards illness good *kammic* effects can arise. The belief in *kamma* also enables us to cope with the painful aspects of life, for example suffering from terminal illness such as leukemia or a more malignant form of cancer with tranquillity and without fruitless struggle, nor negative and depressing mental states. Such acceptance will also enable us to overcome despair, endure the condition to the last days, and thus die a peaceful death.

The emphasis on the kammic cause of health and disease implies individual responsibility for health and illness. *Kamma* is created by choices we made in past lives. Health is to be gained by continuing personal efforts in this life. Good deeds (e.g. regular exercise, proper nutrition, etc.) lead to good health whereas bad deeds (e.g. poor living habits, abusing the body and the mind) in this and previous lives bring illness. The sense of responsibility is much needed in health care. At present, with the invention of "miracle drugs" and the development of new technologies, many people tend to have the illusion that all pain and suffering in life can be eliminated and that all suffering is bad, whether physical, mental, emotional, moral, or spiritual. And by blaming it on external forces people seek external means (e.g. pills, injection, therapies, etc.) of alleviating suffering rather than examining themselves and their own lives and seeking to change what it is within themselves that has resulted in illness. The Buddhist *kamma* view of health and disease, on the contrary, recognizes the reality of self-inflicted disease that can be traced to an individual's own life-style and habits, and encourages one to seek also for the cause of our disease, pain, and suffering within oneself, e.g. in relation to one's own life-styles, decisions, attitudes, and relationships that must be changed. It also recognizes the positive role of disease and suffering in refining our spirit and in strengthening our moral character, e.g. courage, self-understanding, and sympathy towards others.

However, the Buddhist emphasis on *individual kamma* or personal responsibility for health does not mean that Buddhism assigns personal responsibility for all illness. In the Buddhist view *kamma* has both individual and social dimensions. This latter component is what may be termed as *social kamma* which, in health care, refers to the environmental factors that could aggravate or mitigate an *individual kamma*. These factors such as socio-economic factors, e.g. unhealthy and dangerous working conditions, can act as the hazardous/supporting environment for health/illness of an individual. And society could hold employers and businesses responsible if they did not maintain a healthy environment for their workers or provide safety measures. This concept of *social kamma* also implies responsibility on the part of government to provide adequate health care services to all its citizens in proportion to their health needs and medical conditions.

The body and physical health

In the Buddhist perspective the unique body of each of us, both in appearance and structure, is a result of our past *kamma*. The human body is at the same time the means by which we contact the world and the physical manifestation of our mind. Being such an important instrument, the body must be duly attended to, i.e. one must not abuse it through food, alcohol, drugs, or by taxing it with over-indulgence and deprivation. Even enlightenment, the highest goal of Buddhism, cannot be attained by the mortification of the body, as witnessed in the personal experience of the Buddha. This is due to the interdependency of the mind and the body. Intellectual illumination can be attained only when the body is not deprived of anything necessary for the healthy and efficient functioning of all bodily organs.

According to Buddhism, any life lived solely for self-seeking or self-indulgence is a life not worth living. Buddhism therefore encourages us to make use of the body for higher purposes, particularly for attaining the highest goal, *nibbana*, liberation from the endless cycle of birth and rebirth (*samsara*). This can be done by disciplining the body through morality (*sila*) and by mental development through meditation (*bhavana*) focusing on the body, its movements, and traits (e.g. impermanence, insubstantiality, and suffering) as subjects of contemplation. Constant practice of morality and meditation will enable us to have self-control over the appetites, sensations, and egoistic drives.

Physical health is viewed by Buddhism as constituted by the normal functioning of the body and its organically interrelated organs. When one of them fails to function, debility and disease set in. The normal function of the body organs is the result of the harmony and equilibrium of the four primary elements in the body, i.e. earth (*pathavi*), water (*apo*), wind (*vaya*), and fire (*tejo*). If the balance is disturbed, the normal function is disrupted and a state of disease appears. Curing is the restoration of this balance, i.e. putting the entire physical being, and not just the pathologically afflicted part, into good condition. Since each part of the human body is organically related to all other parts, for good health the entire body must be in good condition. In view of the fact that the body, like all phenomena, is always in a state of change, decline, and decay, physical health cannot last long. It is impossible for the body to be perfectly healthy and free from all diseases at all times. Human life is vulnerable to disease at every stage. Disease is a reminder of human fragility. This implies that health is not a totally attainable state. Human wholeness or well-being, therefore, does not mean the absence of all pain and suffering in life, but learning to deal with pain and suffering, how to use it and transcend it for the sake of personal growth and sympathetic understanding of others.

The power of the mind and mental health

Physical health is important because Buddhism regards it to be the means to intellectual enlightenment. Buddhism does not want people to spend a large part of their lives in poor health or else they will not be able to devote themselves to the highest purposes. Although Buddhism views the mind and the body in interdependence, its teaching gives special attention to the mind and its power. It is stated in the very first verse of the Dhammapada that what we are is the result of our thoughts. The source of our lives and hence of our happiness or unhappiness lies within our power. No one can harm us but ourselves. It is the kind of thought we entertain that improves our physical well-being or weakens it, and also ennobles us or degrades us. This is the reason why Buddhism designates thought as the cause of both physical and verbal actions with their *kammic* results and considers mental health of the utmost importance and the training of the mind to attain the highest stage of health as its sole concern. This preoccupation with mental health is also regarded as the true vocation of Buddhist monks. The training is based on the belief that both the body and the mind are prone to sickness. But since the mind is able to detach itself from the body it is possible to have a healthy mind within a sick body.

According to Buddhism for the mind to be healthy, first it is necessary to develop a correct view of the world and ourselves, i.e. a realistic acceptance of the three traits of existence: impermanence, insubstantiality, and suffering of unsatisfactoriness. The adoption of the wrong views makes us see the transitory as permanent, the painful as happy, the impure as pure, and what is not-self as self. Consequently we crave and struggle for what is not – something that does not seem to change, e.g. the illusory permanent and identical self and the permanent object of desire – and we always suffer disappointment. By accepting things as they really are – nothing is permanent and without suffering; the self is in reality nothing more than a name for the complex of psycho-physical elements (*nama-rupa*) – the mind no longer strives for the satisfaction of self-seeking impulses nor clings to objects. As a result the mind is at rest and thereby psychological suffering is eliminated leading to improved mental health.

Apart from changing our thought by the adoption of this correct view and by developing an attitude of detachment towards the world and ourselves, our mental health is dependent on our power to rein in our appetites and to restrain and/or eradicate greed (*lobha*), hatred (*dosa*), anger, and our possessive and aggressive tendencies. All these unwholesome states can act as the cause of mental and physical illness. Such control can be achieved through the practice of morality and meditation. Every set of Buddhist precepts and every type of meditation are aimed at controlling the senses, impulses, and instincts and easing the tension and eliminating the unwholesomeness of thoughts that tend to make the mind sick.

Buddhist meditation is not only a means to cure the mind from its ailments caused by incorrect views, self-indulgence, hatred, and anger of all forms, but is also devised as a means to induce positive wholesome mental states, particularly the four sublime states: loving kindness (*metta*), compassion (*karuna*), sympathetic joy (*mudita*), and equanimity (*upekha*). Loving kindness enables us to love and be kind to one another while compassion wants us to help those in distress. Sympathetic joy is an ability to rejoice in the joy of others and equanimity is the equanimous temperament without being either elated or dejected in the face of the vicissitudes of life – gain and loss, fame and lack of fame, praise and blame, happiness and sorrow. The continual cultivation of these wholesome mental states is an important Buddhist way of making the mind healthy.

Buddhism and Thai health care delivery

In contemporary Thailand both traditional and modern medicine are being used in the provision of health care. But it is the traditional medicine that carries on the Buddhist holistic concept of health focusing on the whole person, while biomedicine is seen as following a narrower concept dissecting human beings into different segments and reducing patient care to the quantifiable control of physical symptoms. Despite this difference the majority of practitioners of these two medical traditions respond with compassion to suffering patients. And compassion is a central Buddhist moral ideal that all are encouraged to practise everywhere and at all times. The ideal is of great importance, particularly in health care where the practitioners are dealing with vulnerable people and have within their power the means to prevent or alleviate further harm or, on the other hand, to permit or cause harm to those already injured. In traditional medicine, compassion is expressed in many ways. For example, the monk-healers usually do not charge for their consultation, and for medications prescribed the cost may be nominal or none at all. In addition these practitioners give adequate time to patients to serve to both their mental and physical needs.

Believing that hospitals are non-profit-seeking institutions erected to serve suffering people, on its part the government expresses the Buddhist central spiritual belief of compassion by requiring its doctors to give free consultation to patients and even free medicine to those who cannot afford to pay. The main problem Thailand is now facing, like other developing nations, is that the available medical resources cannot meet the growing demands of the increasing population. State policy now requires all medical graduates to spend three years in rural areas before working in urban hospitals or setting up their private practice. Among these graduates there are quite a few with keener religious and moral sensitivities, while others are primarily concerned with monetary return. Among those who practise medicine with the Buddhist ideal of compassion, instead of working in the city where they can receive higher incomes and social status, some voluntarily choose to spend their lives with those in dire need, without material rewards. In these cases they are fulfilling the Buddhist higher ideal of compassionate service among suffering fellows. By such service they have stepped beyond the usual human inclination to work in lucrative areas. Dr Soontorn Antarasena and Dr Salyaveth Lekakul, for example, are mobilizing government and private resources to help the rural poor in northeast Thailand who are suffering from diseases of the ear, nose, and throat. They perform free operations where needed and disseminate knowledge for self-care and the prevention of such diseases. To make their services accessible to villagers in different areas, they have set up the first mobile ear, nose, and throat clinic, through which 100,000 patients have been treated and 10,000 operations performed.

Another outstanding example is Dr Pisut Pornsumiritchok who has been working for twelve years at a community hospital in the isolated northern region of Chiengmai, serving the sick and the rural poor. In his treatment of patients, he combines modern medicine with traditional healing, and has a special ward at the hospital to promote traditional herbs and massage in an effort to curb overmedication, such as unnecessary injections and over-utilization of drugs. Dr Pisut is one of the few doctors who sees the danger of overmedicalization and does not want people to spend money unnecessarily for services which go beyond medical needs. He also wants rural people to make more use of indigenous herbs for their ailments. These herbs have been utilized in traditional medicine since the thirteenth century, but have been in decline due to the predominance of Western biomedicine and its "miracle drugs". A resurgence of herbal medicine is necessary to make health care less costly and accessible and affordable to all. One has to commend Dr Pisut for his imaginative efforts to combine Western medicine with traditional medicine to provide effective and co-ordinated health care for Thai people. He has led the way showing how doctors can harmoniously combine biomedicine with traditional treatment.

Because of his concern for the health and well-being of the villagers, Dr Pisut has become involved in many other projects that enhance health. For example, realizing that effective health care goes beyond the hospital's premises, he campaigned for the use of natural pesticides among villagers and initiated community anti-drugs projects in which villagers police their own members. And since the deterioration of the environment also affects health, Dr Pisut became involved in the villagers' community forest conservation efforts. He also participated in the villagers' protest against a lignite mine which had caused severe respiratory illnesses in nearby villages and had increased road deaths due to heavier traffic and the widespread use of amphetamines among mine workers working long hours. In carrying out these activities he is honest and straightforward and, as a result, he has stepped on many influential toes. The lignite mine trucks can no longer pass through many villages. A health official was ousted following Dr Pisut's findings regarding corruption in the villagers' health benefits program. His community anti-drugs business hurts the pockets of village leaders who are in the drug business. His policy of using government AIDS funding to benefit people with the HIV virus and to develop family and community care projects has upset some village leaders and officials who want to use the money for other projects, since the AIDS funds require no financial monitoring. These conflicts of interest have placed him and his family at risk. Yet in spite of these threats, he remains determined to live in rural areas, where the majority of the Thai population lives, to work to enhance the health and well-being of poor villagers, as well as to protect them from the abuses and exploitation brought about by business and bureaucracy.

Buddhist monks, suffering, and compassion

In addition to these doctors, we can also cite health care services provided to the rural poor by Buddhist monks who are motivated solely by the Buddhist ideal of compassion.[2] These monks usually live in rural areas. The benefits of economic development which every Thai government promotes, instead of trickling down to the low-income people, have been widening the gap between the rich and the poor and worsening rural and urban inequality. This inequality is evident in the field of health care. While urban people are enjoying the fruits of progress and prosperity, disease still continues to bring pain and suffering to rural people because of the shortage of health care resources and the inadequacies of basic health care services which these people greatly need. In metropolitan Bangkok, for example, there is a surplus of hospitals and health care providers, whereas the rural areas have scarcely any of them. While affluent people have the choice of health care services, the rural poor who need such services most have little or no access to these resources. When the latter come to the hospitals out of necessity in cities like Bangkok, they have to wait in long queues in crowded corridors to secure brief attention from over-worked medical personnel – who sometimes can be very harsh and impolite to them.

For those whose serious health conditions require the use of modern medical technologies and drugs, the cost becomes almost out of reach, especially when the country does not yet have a general health insurance policy. They may be driven to take out loans or sell land, farm animals, or whatever they own, to meet the costs of medical care, and then have to carry debts for long periods. The tragic part of the situation is that there is no guarantee that they will be cured after all these sacrifices. Because of the high costs and the unpleasant experiences they have had at urban hospitals, the rural poor like to turn to the monks in their areas for local remedies and health care services. After all, Buddhist monks are already known for their social work and compassionate service to the villagers in alleviating their suffering from poverty arising form drought, other natural disasters, landlessness, and indebtedness. Because of their compassion, the monk-healers will never turn suffering people away. Instead they utilize their relevant skills and knowledge gained in their secular lives to effect such relief. In the case of health care, monks who are herbalists usually provide remedies of herbal concoctions combined with religious rituals to the sufferers.

Phrakrudharmadharadhikun of Wat Dharavadee in Nakorn Sridharmarat, southern Thailand, is one of these herbalist-monks. He treats people with broken bones as well as those who suffer from diseases of the bones. In such healing he uses the knowledge of herbal medicine gained from the study of ancient medical texts passed down through the ages. The patients who come for his help are not only from villages in Nakorn Sridharmarat, but also from other provinces, since they do not have enough money to meet the cost of healing at hospitals. Health care given by the monk is accessible, available at all times, and free, without any solicitation for donations. When asked about his dedicated work the monk said:

> I am very glad to be able to help people and to make myself available to them at all times. I am not tired of this work even if there are too many patients each day. I have no special office because I like to sit where people can find me easily. I always treat the patients impartially, wanting to restore health to all of them. I am providing them not only with free services but also with simple food and lodging when needed and available since these people are poor. Even though some advised me to keep a record of their names and addresses so that when donations are needed the temple may contact them, I refused to do so. This is because as a Buddhist monk I am obliged to help all those who are suffering. Actually the poor villagers have been providing me with food and other necessities. So why should I ask them to pay for the cost of healing? Besides, the lodging and food that I give them here, when available, are very simple in comparison with what hospitals are offering. People also like to come here with their necessities such as mats, mosquito nets, a pot and a pan. I do not want them to feel obligated to give something back to the temple in return. They already spent money on bus or boat fares. And I do not want them to spend more for donations. Of course, if I asked them for donations certainly they would have to borrow money for such donations, and as a result be burdened with debts. That is the underlying reason why I do not want to ask their names and addresses. For me they are just suffering people who need help, and I am very glad to be helpful to them.

As a result of the compassionate work of this monk, patients receiving treatment at the temple also have the impulse to share. One boy who worked as a spare on a truck came from a poor village in one of the southern provinces. He related his feelings and experiences after falling from a truck and breaking his hip and leg. He said:

> I did not have enough money to go to the hospital in the city. I went first to a private clinic where the doctor asked me whether I could pay for the treatment. I said I could not because I have no father and my widowed mother cannot work. When the doctor knew that I did not have enough money he was reluctant to treat me. I came to the temple on the advice of some friends. Here I am receiving treatment free of charge. And my mother can also be with me and cook for me. Luang Poh (the monk) never asked for my name. He only wanted to know the cause of my pain and suffering. He visits me each day both in the morning and evening. At the beginning when my mother took me here I could not move my body. But now I can move it, though slowly, and I am sure that very soon I will be all right. If I had gone to the hospital my mother would have had to borrow money, and it would take months for us to repay. Here Luang Poh does not ask for any money at all and I am very happy to be here.

Another patient, a girl from a different province, fell from her house, which is built on stilts, and suffered a bone fracture that makes walking a painful experience. She is also poor, with no father and a mother who lives from hand to mouth. When asked about the reason for coming to the temple the girl said:

> My mother could not take me to the hospital as we have no money. We cannot borrow money from our relatives as they also are poor. Here at the temple there is no need for us to pay for the treatment. I am now recovering through the help of Luang Poh.

The view of this patient is typical of others who seek help from the temple because they cannot afford the cost of health care services at hospitals and clinics. It is also very easy for the patients to meet the monk because he is always at the temple to attend to their needs. Even though it is usual for the lay Buddhist to pay respect to the monk by addressing him with special language, the monk does not require any ceremony at all. He only wants to know the cause and nature of the pain, so that he can give the appropriate treatment.

There are many similar monks in other provinces around the country who, out of compassion, use their knowledge of herbal medicine to take care of poor sick people without any charge or for a nominal fee. Most of their patients are cured and treatments are quite successful. Many of the diseases monks treat are those which rural people regularly suffer, such as respiratory diseases, bone fractures, allergies, glaucoma, ulcers, high blood pressure, diabetes, back pain, and snake bites. Treatments usually consist of herbal concoctions combined with religious rituals and the practice of meditation. Some monks, such as Phra Lek Pabhasara of Wat Klongsam in Pathumdhain, even treat cancer patients. A few of these cases have been successfully treated, with the disease controlled or eliminated altogether. Even some doctors from hospitals recommended that their cancer patients in the last stage to go to the temple for humane health care. In such cases the patients are taught to practise mindful meditation to cope with pain and to calm the mind and ultimately to accept death in tranquillity. They are also provided with an opportunity to make merit to ensure a good rebirth.

Apart from cancer, another deadly disease in Thailand is AIDS. The Ministry of Public Health estimates that the number of Thais infected with the HIV virus is 750,000 – nearly 20,000 of whom have developed full-blown AIDS. The problem AIDS patients have been encountering is that the government cannot provide adequate health care for them. An additional problem is that many health care personnel and members of the general public have hostile attitudes towards these sufferers. Accordingly, AIDS patients may find it difficult to procure treatment at hospitals, and their families and friends may shun them. In addition, when their infection is discovered, their employers usually dismiss them. Such experiences of rejection make these AIDS sufferers very sad, some becoming depressed to the point of wanting to end their lives, or some reacting aggressively by intentionally seeking to spread the deadly virus.

Like the rural poor we have discussed, AIDS sufferers usually turn to the temples as the last resort. The monks, unlike lay people, cannot turn their backs on these sufferers, and try their best to find ways and means to help them. For example, Phra Preecha of Wat Tam Sriwilai in Saraburi near Bangkok uses special herbal concoctions to boost the patient's immune system to resist the virus. The herbs numbering thirty and used in these concoctions cannot be bought from the indigenous drug stores but have to be collected in the deep jungle. Along with herbal treatments, the monk prescribes a vegetarian diet, exercise, merit-making (such as helping others and observance of the precepts), and the practice of mindful meditation. Merit-making and meditation are components of the healing process because the monk believes that healing is related to spirituality and that religious life can help healing. Through merit-making the patient develops an ability to "give" while meditation enables him/her to develop self-control and to let go of stresses caused by anger and anxiety. This compassionate work of the monk is appreciated by all AIDS sufferers who are being cared for. One patient recalled,

> When I knew that I had AIDS, I decided to hang myself in a park. I did not want to come to a slow and undignified end. But the taxi driver who drove me to the park, suspecting my intention, did not leave me alone. He stayed with me, consoled me, and finally drove me to this temple for no fare. I am felling better now. The taxi driver and Luang Phor have saved my life. I am determined to stay with Luang Phor to help other sufferers.

Though this particular treatment is still experimental there are at least two specific cases out of one hundred AIDS patients in the earlier stages who have been declared by hospital doctors to be completely cured. Other patients remain asymptomatic and either stabilize or increase their T-cells. Consequently, a large number of patients have come to the temple to seek help from the monk who, in the absence of any government support, is quite over-burdened, particularly when the resources of the temple are very limited. The monk has only two voluntary assistants and he himself has not enough time to rest, having to treat the patients from dawn to dusk. This raises the question of the limits of compassion for the monk. He says,

> I am very tired and my health is deteriorating. At times while treating patients I have to rush to my lodging to throw up because of over-work and exhaustion. But I have great sympathy for these sufferers who have no other places to go, so of course, I treat them free of charge. But some of their relatives like to donate money to the temple. This enables me to buy more herbs from villagers and to help more patients. Since the temple has very limited space, I like to advise people to take the medicine home and to come back only if there is no improvement. If they follow my advice on diet, life-style, merit-making, and meditation while taking the prescribed herbal con-coctions, I expect the cure to be effected in one year and a half. Apart from treatment I encourage all patients to have hope instead of despair otherwise their conditions will become worse. It is not important for me at all to know how they got AIDS and whether they are good people or not. All I know is that they are in great suffering and I have to help to relieve their suffering.

Wat Tam Sriwilai treats only AIDS patients in the earlier, curable, stages. There is another temple which takes care of those in the full-blown stages where no cure is possible. This temple is Wat Prabat Namphu in Lopburi, another province near Bangkok, and the monk is Phra Alongkot. Moved by compassion for those AIDS sufferers who have nowhere to go for needed care, the monk has transformed his small temple into a hospice. Without professional knowledge about AIDS, he wears no protective clothes when treating these patients. When AIDS patients were initially accepted into the temple, other monks fled and villagers threatened to stop supporting the temple because of their fear of AIDS. Lacking proper knowledge about this deadly disease the villagers believed (wrongly) that the disease could be spread easily (e.g. through mosquito bites) and, as a preventive measure, demanded that the monk keep the patients under mosquito nets at all times. During this period, Phra Alongkot had to deal with the hostile attitudes of the villagers as well as procure adequate resources in order to provide proper health care for the AIDS patients. After three years of hard work he managed to persuade the villagers to develop compassion for these patients and to support the temple's humanitarian work. Gradually the villagers began to follow him – even visiting the patients and helping to treat them. The treatment consisted mostly of traditional herbs, diet, and meditation. Apart from the medicinal treatment, patients are encouraged to form a support group and to enjoy life, however short it may be. At present the temple has five volunteers from the villages.

The monk is now receiving increasing assistance, including financial support from NGOs and the general public. Government agencies are also encouraging other temples to follow the example of Wat Prabat Namphu. Even though the monk cannot cure the patients, the temple is a refuge for patients in their final days. At the temple they are supported and cared for without any charge, and often live longer. When they do pass away they let go of their lives peacefully. The provision of free health care adds a burden for the temple, however. Few relatives visit the temple and when the patients die, their bodies are cremated and their bones kept at the temple because relatives will not receive them for fear of contracting HIV. The Ministry of Public Health and some NGOs are at present assisting the temple to initiate a home care project for AIDS sufferers which will establish a supportive community for them. To implement this project, Phra Alongkot has to work harder to persuade people in different villages to take care of AIDS patients in their own areas and not to bring them to the temple. It is not important whether he succeeds or not, for he has already set an example of translating the high ideal of Buddhism into practice, and has contributed, though in a limited way, towards the alleviation of suffering in contemporary Thai society. When divorced from action, the moral ideal of compassion is nothing at all.

We must also take note of other forms of Buddhist compassion in action. There are numerous monks who live and work for others, but who are not herbalists. They are involved in providing health care to suffering people through other means, such as establishing hospitals and health clinics in needy rural areas. These monks usually command respect of lay Buddhists because of their moral perfection and exemplary lives. Since it is believed that making merit to these monks yields the highest merit, lay people like to give large donations to them. Instead of utilizing the donated funds to enlarge their temples, the monks build hospitals or clinics in needy rural areas, or support existing hospitals to enable them to extend medical services to the needy. One of these monks is Phra Maha Bua of Wat Pa Ban Tat,

Udondhani Province. He gives millions of donated money each year to provide mobile units and additional equipment necessary to increase health care services to needy patients in state hospitals which suffer from inadequate budgets.

The abbot of Wat Rai Khing, Phra Mahaviranuwat, in Nakorn Pathom, south of Bangkok, is another notable example of a selfless monk. In earlier years, people in the temple district had no health clinics in their neighbourhood. They went to Bangkok for needed health care services when necessary. For many years the district officials asked the Ministry of Public Health to build a clinic there, but without any result. The abbot saw the need and took the initiative to ask for public donations. As one having great respect from people not only in the area but throughout the country large donations flowed in, and instead of a modest clinic he built a hospital of 130 beds on the temple grounds with the approval of the Ministry of Public Health. The name of the hospital is "Meta Prajaraksa Hospital" which means "The Hospital of Loving Kindness for Healing People". To avoid the hospital being an ongoing financial burden to the temple, he gave the hospital to the King who handed it over to the Ministry of Public Health. The hospital is now staffed by personnel provided by the Ministry and is serving people from different villages. For those patients who cannot pay for treatment, the temple underwrites the bills. The abbot also established a special foundation to support the hospital to render free medical services to monks and needy people, as well as to purchase medical equipment when the government budgetary allocation is insufficient. The abbot has also used temple donations to support secular schools in the district by providing them with modern equipment such as language learning facilities and computers. Donations are further used to provide scholarships for students from poor families to further their studies at institutes of higher learning.

The work of Phra Maha Bua and the abbot of Wat Rai Khing are examples of compassionate services provided by Buddhist monks to the community. Instead of just "receiving", they use donations to contribute to the health and well-being of the villagers. By so doing, they reinterpret Buddhism and its role in society. Their selfless work helps make Buddhism more relevant and appealing to members of the new generation who look to religion for active contribution to both the spiritual and material development of the community. Seeing the social benefit of their donations, the rich become more conscious of the need to use their resources to help the poor, while those benefiting from such contributions live with hope as they realize that they are not neglected and left to their own destiny by themselves. This is the reason why people continue to make donations to these two monks. The more the monks "give", the more donations they "receive". While the personality and compassion of these monks generate much generosity among their followers, there is also a concern that this outflow of generosity may not last once the monks pass away. We can only hope that such compassion will continue in the days to come, especially when the conscience of the rich has been touched by the selfless work of the monks and by the manifest fruits of their work.

Conclusion

In Thai culture, Buddhist ideas and values have a strong impact on the understanding of health and the approach to health care. The Buddhist concept of health has a significant influence on traditional Thai medicine in its holistic approach to health care focusing on the entire person. This leads to the adoption of the Buddhist ideal of compassion as the guiding principle. Health care is to be given to all patients with loving kindness. This ideal is also upheld by some of the practitioners of modern medicine as can be seen among those who serve the rural poor, having only their benefit in mind.

The practice of Buddhist compassion is more fully manifested by the Buddhist monks. Their approaches give due importance to the spiritual dimension of the patient, which is lacking in modern medicine, through emphasis on religious commitment and practices as another important factor in the restoration of health. To this end meditation is added to provide the patients with the mind–body relaxation techniques and to enable them to develop wholesome mental states which have great effects on physical health. This way the monks are giving the patients more complete healing and not mere treatments.

There is no doubt that in a time when there are grave imbalances in the allocation of health care resources and unnecessary persistence in inadequacies in basic health care services, these monks play an important role in enhancing the lives of the poor and the disadvantaged in the remote areas of the country by relieving their suffering and restoring their health. This is a way of bringing justice to poor people who are unduly neglected. It is also a way of helping them to have lives with a significant religious meaning, free from the suffering caused by illness and disease.

Notes

1. This law is also referred to as the law of causality according to which a deed is likened to a seed which will sooner or later result in certain fruits.

2. All data about the work of these monks were collected in the field during 1995-1996. See also Pinit Ratanakul (1990) "The Dynamic of Tradition and Change in Theravade Buddhism", in *Development, Modernization, and Tradition in Southeast Asia: Lessons from Thailand,* ed. Pinit Ratanakul and U. Kyan Than, Bangkok, Mahidol University.

Chapter 3
Concepts of Health and Disease in Traditional Chinese Medicine

Edwin Hui

Prior to 1840, "traditional Chinese medicine"[1] was the only medical system being practised in China for both acute and chronic diseases. Grounded on traditional philosophy, especially cosmology, traditional Chinese medicine was developed into a highly sophisticated theoretical system which directs its clinical application in therapeutic regimens such as acupuncture and Chinese herbal medicine. Modern biomedicine was not introduced in China to any significant extent until after the Opium War in 1841 and since then both medical systems have existed rather uneasily together in China. Between 1840 and 1954, there was a tendency for the Western medical system to be dominant, and traditional Chinese medicine was treated as an inferior system. In fact, in 1929 the then nationalist government even considered a legislative initiative to outlaw traditional Chinese medicine. It was only due to the severe opposition from the practitioners of traditional Chinese medicine that the law was not passed.

In 1954 the current regime, the People's Republic of China (PRC), saw the need to rehabilitate and revitalize traditional Chinese medicine, which has since enjoyed an unprecedented popularity due to governmental support. Since Mao Tse-tung declared that "Chinese Medicine is a great treasure house! We must make all efforts to uncover it and raise its standards!" (Unschuld 1985, 251), many traditional Chinese medicine hospitals, schools, research centres, and herbal pharmaceutical factories have been built. The total percentage of health care personnel directly involved in traditional Chinese medicine has been reported to be in the neighbourhood of 17–22 percent. So much so that in 1982 the development of traditional Chinese medicine and modern biomedicine were written together in the constitution of PRC. Currently in China, about 60 percent of all therapeutic interventions can be classified as Western biomedical and the remaining 40 percent employ a combined Western–traditional Chinese medicine approach. Studies have indicated that the therapeutic efficacy has been the same. Because of the employment of traditional Chinese medicine, the cost of medical service is greatly reduced, and is currently occupying roughly 3 percent of total national income (Lu 1995, 117).

The concept of holism in traditional Chinese medicine

Holism is a fundamental characteristic of traditional Chinese medicine. A human person is not viewed in fragments as body, soul, and spirit. These categories have been available since ancient times in China, but as an integrated whole. The concept of health is accordingly conceived holistically. Furthermore, since human beings are considered products of nature, humanity and its natural environment are inseparably and interdependently related. Ancient Chinese medicine, as represented by the author(s) of "The Yellow Emperor's Classic of Internal Medicine" (YECIM), held that humanity and the universe together constitute one "holistic" entity and humans and their health are therefore conditioned and affected by changes that occur in the natural (cosmic) environment. In other words, traditional Chinese medicine and traditional Chinese philosophy see both the human person and the person–nature dyad as holistic entities, and maintaining the integrity of these two holistic entities is a fundamental factor in the maintenance of a person's health.

The Chinese understanding of nature and the cosmos is expressed in three important philosophical concepts: *ch'i* (material or vital force), "*yin* and *yang*", and *wu-hsing* (five elements). Because these overlapping and intertwining concepts are employed to understand and explain humanity and the cosmos we inhabit, the conceptualization of health is also framed and formulated by these complex philosophical and epistemic paradigms. In order to understand health in the traditional Chinese medicine formulation of it, we will briefly describe these three philosophical concepts and their applications to the Chinese understanding of the human body and of health.

The concept of ch'i [2] *(material force, energy, vital or life-giving force, steam)*

Ancient Chinese philosophers and medical practitioners derived the concept of *ch'i* from empirical observations of the behaviour of physical matter and of human beings in health and disease. In the context of traditional Chinese medicine, *ch'i* is an objective reality which is accessible to human senses; for example, practitioners of traditional Chinese medicine believe that the movements of *ch'i* can be detected by feeling or even by visual observation. *Ch'i* is derived from and connected to visible physical matter, and every physical object in the universe is believed to have its own particular *ch'i*. The cosmos has its own *ch'i*, which is manifested in and detectable through the various meteorological changes such as cold, heat, humidity, wind, rain, dryness, etc. A human person has more than one kind of *ch'i* because of the different visceral organs, and the most important one is "*yuan ch'i*" (the primal vital energy) which relates to the process of procreation (the male sperm). Because each physical object is associated with its own *ch'i*, it becomes the medium of communication between various physical entities. The *ch'i* of the cosmos connects with the human person and various organs of the body, making it possible for the human person–cosmos to be seen as a holistic entity. In the YECIM's "Treatise on the Communication of the Force of Life with Heaven" the Yellow Emperor is quoted as saying,

> From earliest times the communication with Heaven has been the very foundation of life; this foundation exists between *Yin* and *Yang* and between Heaven and Earth and within the six points [which are the four points of the compass, the Zenith and the Nadir]. The (heavenly) breath [*ch'i*] prevails in the nine divisions, in the nine orifices, in the five viscera, and in the twelve joints; they are all pervaded by the breath of Heaven. (Huang Ti 1907, 105)

Not only the cosmos connects with the human beings through the *ch'i* of heaven, the various organs within the human body also communicate with each other through their respective *ch'i* and thereby affect each other. "The five viscera are in communication with one another and influence one another" (Huang Ti 1907, 179). Traditional Chinese medicine identifies twelve main vessels in the human body which essentially are channels through which the different *ch'i* move, and one of the main causes of the disease state is obstructions of the flow of *ch'i* in the body. Health implies that the *ch'i* between the organs of the person are flowing normally as detected by the pulses of the body.

The concept of yin–yang[3]

The importance of the notion of the interaction of *yin* and *yang* in traditional Chinese medicine can be seen in an opening remark of chapter 5 in the YECIM, which says that "The principle of *yin* and *yang* [the male and the female elements in nature] is the basic principle of the entire universe. It is the principle of everything in creation ... it is the root and source of life and death;" (Huang Ti 1970, 115). The ancient Chinese concept of *yin* and *yang*, which first appeared in Chinese philosophical writings in the mid-Chou dynasty (1111-249 BCE), is a dialectical concept attempting to explain various phenomena of the universe which often appear to be at one and the same time interdependent on and in opposition to each other. The dialectic of *yin* and *yang* seeks to understand the fundamental rules and rhythms of such seemingly contradictory operations and developments in nature. It is believed that all natural events in the universe operate according to the dialectic of *yin* and *yang*. As YECIM states, "Heaven was created by an accumulation of *yang*, the element of light; Earth was created by an accumulation of *yin*, the element of darkness" (Huang Ti 1970, 115). "*Yin* and *yang* create desires and vigour in men and women. The ways of *yin* and *yang* are to the left and to the right. Water and fire are the evidences and symbols of *yin* and *yang*. *Yin* and *yang* are the source of power and the beginning of everything in creation" (Huang Ti 1970, 120). Accordingly, as the ultimate unit of matter and the vital force, *ch'i* also operates dialectically in the *yin–yang* fashion, regardless whether the *ch'i* derives from the cosmos or human sources.

At the risk of oversimplification, the dialectic of *yin* and *yang* can be understood to operate in four distinct ways. In the first place, *yin* and *yang* operate in opposition to each other to reach a state of dynamic equilibrium. The regularities of the four seasons are examples of such a balance, the disturbance of which will lead to seasonal irregularities, such as excessive dryness when *yang* gets the upper hand. Human body functions also follow this pattern. "If *yin* is not equal to *yang*, then the pulse becomes weak and sickly and causes madness. If *yang* is not equal to *yin*, then the breaths [*ch'i*] which are contained in the five viscera will conflict with each other and the circulation ceases" (Huang Ti 1970, 108). Secondly, *yin* and *yang* are mutually dependent on each other and co-operate with each other for efficient functioning.

In the human body, *ch'i* is supposed to have affinity with *yang* and blood is associated with *yin*, and the YECIM teaches that *ch'i* is the "commander" of blood whereas blood is the "mother" of *ch'i*, indicating that *yin* and *yang* are intimately related to and dependent on each other. Finally, *yin* and *yang* may be mutually transformative. This takes place when imbalance occurs in the extreme degree and one state far exceeds the other quantitatively, so that the YECIM could say that "the state of extreme coldness [*yin*] leads to heat [*yang*], and the state of extreme heat leads to coldness". Through mutual dependency and transformation, *yin* and *yang* are maintained in harmony. All bodily functions are the result of the harmony of *yin* and *yang*; a mild imbalance implies a diseased state, and a total disruption of the harmony would lead to the ending of the holistic life entity. "If *yang* accumulates excessively, one will die from the (resulting) disease." (Huang Ti 1970, 107) "If *yin* is in a state of tranquillity and *yang* is preserved perfectly, then one's spirit is in perfect order. If *yin* and *yang* separate, one's essence and vital force will be destroyed." (Huang Ti 1970, 109)

The theory of the five phases/elements

The concept of *yin* and *yang*, in order to be applied to real natural phenomena, must be concretized into more tangible components. And this is expressed in the theory of the five phases/elements, which are metal, wood, water, fire, and earth. The theory of the five phases/elements can be viewed as the natural science version of the metaphysical concept of *yin* and *yang*. The five elements are fundamental categories of all matter in the universe, which derive their operative, developmental, and interactive patterns according to the dynamic cycles of subjugation and generation among the five phases/elements. YECIM explains that

> when the element of wood reaches the element of metal it is felled; when the element of fire reaches the element of water it will be extinguished; when the element of the earth is reached by the element of wood it is penetrated; when the element of metal reaches the element of fire it is dissolved; and when water reaches the earth its flow is interrupted and cut off" (Huang Ti 1970, 215).

Thus, metal subjugates wood, water subjugates fire, wood subjugates earth, fire subjugates metal, and earth subjugates water. The sequence of generation is: metal creates water, water creates wood, wood creates fire, fire creates earth, and earth creates metal. As an example of the application of the theory of the five phases/elements to events of nature, these five phases/elements are said to be "distributed" or attached over the seasons so that spring belongs to wood, summer belongs to fire, late summer belongs to earth, fall belongs to metal, and winter belongs to water. Since the human body is part of nature, the five phases/elements are also distributed to the five most important internal organs of the body which determine the functions of all the other parts of the body and emotions. In this manner, the liver is assigned to wood, heart to fire, spleen to earth, lungs to metal, and kidneys to water. In fact, the Chinese theory of five phases/elements assigns the five elemental attributes to every observable object and phenomenon in the universe, from seasons, climatic conditions, animals, grains, human organs, tissues, orifices, emotions, to flavour, odour, sand, colour, music, direction, and planets. It becomes apparent that through this system of five phases/elements, traditional Chinese medicine was not only able to explain the various interactions between the body organs, but also the influence of environmental factors (seasons, weather, etc.) on the human body and emotions. And because the internal organs possess their own sound, colour, odour, and flavour, which traditional Chinese medicine believes are accessible to human senses, the theory of five phases/elements has significant roles in the assessment of health and diagnosis and prognostication of diseases as well.

Health and disease in traditional Chinese medicine

From the perspective of traditional Chinese medicine, a person enjoys perfect health when s/he has a strong and unobstructed flow of *ch'i*, is under the influence of well-balanced *yin–yang* forces, and is accompanied by a harmony with the five phases/elements of the environment. In that state of *zheng ch'i* (literally, vital energy) "pathogenic factors" will not be able to interfere with the health of the person and health is maintained. But when the *yin–yang* forces are out of balance and the operation of the five phases/elements has been disrupted by the seasons or the weather conditions, then the *ch'i* of the human body is said to have been weakened, allowing the "pathogenic factors" to cause the diseased state. In other words, the state of health is a state of equilibrium between the *zheng ch'i* of the body and "pathogenic factors". In ancient traditional Chinese medicine, these "pathogenic factors" are ill-defined; they may be external to the body in the form of weather irregularities (excessive cold or heat) or inside the person in the form of emotional upheavals (anger, bereavement, etc.). But regardless how ill-defined these pathogenic factors may be, they are believed to be objective entities or realities, which traditional Chinese medicine collectively refer to as "*xie*", which literally means evil. In other words, health is the proper functioning of human physiology which lends to our body resistance sufficient strength to gain an upper hand over the pathogenic processes which are almost always present.

It is important to realize that according to traditional Chinese medicine, to maintain health as well as to fight off pathogenic processes, the focus is primarily on the maintenance and promotion of the *zheng ch'i* (building up body resistance) and only secondarily on the pathogenic factors. Traditional Chinese medicine holds the view that if the *zheng ch'i* (body resistance) is good or strong, pathogenic processes will not be able to gain entrance into the body or, even if they gain entrance, they will be controlled by the *zheng ch'i* so that the disease state will not emerge. For this reason, traditional Chinese medicine emphasizes preventive medicine and health maintenance, with therapeutic intervention to dispel pathogenic factors reserved only for acute conditions. Even for acute conditions, health maintenance procedures (i.e. measures to strengthen resistance) are usually implemented simultaneously. YECIM states that, "Hence the sages did not treat those who were already ill; they instructed those who were not yet ill. ...To administer medicines to diseases which have already developed ... is comparable to the behaviour of those persons who begin to dig a well after they have become thirsty ... Would these actions not be too late?" (Huang Ti 1970, 105).

Health maintenance

Since health means the *zheng ch'i* in the body gaining an upper hand over pathogenic factors, to maintain health is to maintain and promote *zheng ch'i*. In this regard three things are emphasized: (i) maintenance of internal balance, (ii) employment of exercise, massage, and "therapeutic diet", (iii) life-style arrangements and practices.

(i) The maintenance of internal balance is grounded on the concept of *yin* and *yang*. Traditional Chinese medicine rooted in "YECIM" teaches that body structures are under the influence of *yang* forces, while body functions are represented by *yin* forces. Since *yin* and *yang* forces are interrelated, this provides the theoretical basis for the relationship between structure and function in traditional Chinese medicine. Health can therefore be achieved if the *yin* and *yang* forces, which pervade all the organs and functions of the body, are in balance and harmony. And this balance of *yin* and *yang* can only be achieved when the body is considered holistically. In this regard traditional Chinese medicine emphasizes the interconnection and communication between different solid viscera, hollow organs, vessels, and joints – mediated by the *ch'i* of these respective organs.

(ii) Traditional Chinese medicine believes that the maintenance of internal balance can be greatly assisted by various exercises such as "*qigong*" and "*taiji*" which involve an integration of body movements and breathing exercises, and relaxation of the mind. Over the last two millennia, traditional Chinese medicine has also developed very elaborate massage techniques to maintain the flow of *ch'i* in the body. Traditional Chinese medicine also emphasizes usage of various "medicines" for health maintenance purposes. They may therefore be considered as a form of "therapeutic diet". The "medicines" may include herbs, metals, and animal organs. It is believed that when used properly, especially in a way consistent with the seasons which are related with the "five phases/elements", these medicines are of utmost use to strengthen the *ch'i* of the person and maintain health.

(iii) Finally, the holistic concept of health in terms of a person's harmonious relation with the environment is seen in traditional Chinese medicine's emphasis on life-style arrangements and practices. This is reflected in the emphasis on "self mental care", attention to dietary care, living environment (e.g. the location of one's home and stewardship of one's land), and meticulous adjustment to changes of the four seasons. By its concern with self mental care, traditional Chinese medicine acknowledges the importance of the mental, emotional, and spiritual aspects of a person towards health maintenance. In that context, traditional Chinese medicine's mental care includes the teaching against aggressive pursuit of personal wealth and success, which traditional Chinese medicine believes would add to one's emotional burden, leading to anxiety, fear, and depression. Traditional Chinese medicine advises people to pursue a life of simplicity and ordinariness as a way to good health. This teaching of self mental care has been influenced by Daoism and Buddhism. Traditional Chinese medicine also recommends that one should curb one's sexual desire and cultivate personal moral virtue, believing that excessive and promiscuous sexual activity is definitely harmful to health, particularly by weakening the primordial *yuan ch'i* in the body, which is related to procreation. Because traditional Chinese medicine believes that food, like medicines, can be classified into different natures according to the theories of *yin–yang* and five phases/elements (e.g. cold, heat, dry, wet, etc.), it is recommended that different dietary regimens should be followed for different kinds of deficiencies detected in the person in order to maintain the balance of *yin–yang* and health. For example, in a menstruating woman because of the loss of blood, the influence of *yang* force is decreased and cold food which belongs to the realm of the *yin* force must be avoided.

Traditional Chinese medicine also believes that living environments are intimately related to one's health, so that location, direction, elevation are all important factors influencing one's health. This is largely due to the belief that the five phases/elements of the environment have direct impact on the bodily organs and functions. This is particularly obvious in traditional Chinese medicine's emphasis on the relation between climatic and seasonal changes and human health. The YECIM states that "In order to bring into harmony the human body one takes as standard the laws of the four seasons and the five phases/elements" (Huang Ti 1970, 198). That is because human lives are supposed to be dependent on the *ch'i* of the cosmos. The season of spring is considered "the period of the beginning and development (of life). The breaths [*ch'i*] of Heaven and Earth are prepared to give birth; thus everything is developing and flourishing" (Huang Ti 1970, 102). To assimilate these breaths of spring life, the YECIM continues to recommend that "After a night of sleep people should get up early (in the morning); they should walk briskly around the yard; they should loosen their hair and slow down their movements (body); by these means they can (fulfil) their wish healthfully" (Huang Ti 1970, 102). Correspondingly, there is a set of dietary menus more appropriate for spring and this may include fresh fruits and vegetables and other produce from the soil. In contrast, the winter is considered

> the period of closing and storing ... People should retire early at night and rise late in the morning ... They should suppress and conceal their wishes ... as though they had been fulfilled ... All this is in harmony with the atmosphere of winter and all this is the method for the protection of one's storing." (Huang Ti 1970, 103)

In terms of food, items that fall within the *yang* categories, such as meat and wine, considered to be particularly useful for re-enforcement of *ch'i* and blood of the body, are recommended for winter. We can see that maintenance of health is a matter of living a life closely integrated with one's environment. As YECIM states unequivocally, "Those who rebel against the basic rules of the universe sever their own roots and ruin their selves" (Huang Ti 1970, 104) and this includes obeying the principles of *yin* and *yang* and the five phases/elements, as well as conforming to the changes of the four seasons. "*Yin* and *yang*, the two principles in nature, and the four seasons are the beginning and the end of everything and they are also the cause of life and death." (Huang Ti 1970, 105)

Personal and social responsibility in traditional Chinese medicine

From the perspective of traditional Chinese medicine, health and disease are ultimately a matter of balance and imbalance. Because traditional Chinese medicine holds a holistic view of health and disease, balance and imbalance have both internal and external dimensions. The internal dimension calls for proper cultivation of character and adoption of a proper diet and life-style in order that one's internal dynamic health force can be developed. In this regard, personal responsibility is emphasized. But the external dimension of balance and imbalance include social and environmental dimensions which require a communal involvement. In this sense, traditional Chinese medicine is conscious of the importance of social responsibility in health maintenance and disease prevention.

Under the predominantly Confucian influence, Chinese society is a hierarchically arranged, family based society in which interpersonal relations are meticulously defined and carefully differentiated in order that people may treat each other with the appropriate attitudes and affections – for example, filial piety (for children towards parents), respect (for younger siblings towards older siblings), faithfulness (for inferior towards superiors), and altruism (between equals). Cultivation of these virtues is carried out in a social context and for the purpose of fulfilling social responsibility. Traditional Chinese medicine firmly believes that social harmony is essential for the maintenance of emotional and mental health and traditional Chinese medicine holds the belief that there is a direct causal relationship between moral uprightness and physical illness, which is often perceived as affected by "unfilial behaviour or other breakdown in interpersonal relations" (Klein-man et al. 1975, 274). For this reason, interpersonal behaviours are strictly enforced through a code of propriety in traditional Chinese society and this is done not only for the purpose of social harmony, but ultimately also for the purpose of health maintenance. A person who refuses to abide by the socially sanctioned norm will be ostracized or expelled from the family/community because s/he will be perceived as a threat to the well-being of members of the community.

Similarly, the importance of social responsibility in health maintenance is also seen in the Chinese people's concern with architecture and land use. Because living environments are believed to be intimately related to health and disease, in a traditional Chinese community, the configuration, location, and situation of houses, burial sites, roads, farms, etc. are matters of communal concern. For example, no one individual can arbitrarily plant or cut down a tree without the consensual approval of all members of a community who may be affected by the presence or absence of a tree. Burial sites are notorious as a source of dispute in traditional Chinese communities because it is believed that where one's ancestor(s) is (are) buried has direct bearing on the physical well-being of members of the community.

While the role of personal and social responsibilities can reasonably be delineated in health maintenance in traditional Chinese medicine, the same cannot be said for health care where the latter is defined more in terms of intervention in disease and restoration of lost health. Before the introduction of modern biomedicine, outside the urban areas in the more confined communities or villages each with no more than one or two thousand people, it was a usual practice for a community to retain the service of a practitioner of traditional Chinese medicine who lived among the people of the community. His expected primary role of maintaining health rather than curing disease can be seen by the fact that the practitioner was usually paid when everyone was healthy; but in the event of a massive breakdown of health, the practitioner might be blamed for not doing his job, his salary might be withheld and he might even be fired (just as local gods can be replaced if people are dissatisfied with their services). Because the Chinese people, even in modern times, are still so deeply influenced by the holistic biopsychosocial paradigm of health, it is interesting to note that in a national conference on medical ethics held in 1995, with the theme of "The goal of medicine", the overwhelming majority of the participants were of the opinion that health maintenance should still be the goal of twenty-first century Chinese medicine. Most participants found in the WHO definition an affirmation of the traditional Chinese medical paradigm. Many of the presenters in the Conference urged that the allocation of the limited resources should favour preventive medicine, public health, population control, education on health maintenance, and physical conditioning over high-tech modern medicine which is seen to benefit only a minority of people.

Relation of the traditional Chinese medicine to modern practices of medicine in China

Experiences in the West, particularly in North America where 11–14 percent of GNP is being spent on health care utilizing modern "high-tech" biomedicine, have alerted the Chinese people to the need of supplementing modern Western-style medicine with traditional Chinese medicine. In a survey done in the city of Dalian in China in 1995, 40.6 percent of a group of 500 health care personnel believed that traditional Chinese medicine has decisive significance for health care in China; 46.0 percent indicated that traditional Chinese medicine is important though not necessarily decisive; and only 8 percent felt that traditional Chinese medicine is not important. Similar patterns of response were elicited from patients, patients' family members, as well as a cross-section of the public not immediately involved in a medical encounter. In fact, these last three groups score 6–16 percentage points higher than the health care personnel group in considering traditional Chinese medicine as a decisive factor for medical care in China, and 3–5 percentage points lower in believing that traditional Chinese medicine is unimportant (Su et al. 1995). So, with the implementation of the program of modernization in China since the 1980s, what we witness in this part of the world is a rather interesting although at times uneasy scenario. While most people continue to make it a personal responsibility to practise preventive medicine in the form of health maintenance along the traditional Chinese medicine model, an increasingly large number of people, especially the city dwellers, have come to appreciate the efficacy of modern biomedicine, which has been subjected to a market-economy model. And all of this is taking place when the country officially continues to embrace a Marxist ideology, which considers health care to be a state affair.

In Taiwan, where Western medicine is more dominant than in Mainland

China, a survey was done in 1990 in which 79 percent of respondents regarded traditional Chinese medicine as more effective in treating the "root" of disease (Chi 1994, 314). Survey data also support the view that in Taiwan, even though less than one-third of the population actually consults a licensed traditional Chinese medicine practitioner, the number of people who use traditional Chinese medicine in other forms such as self-medication or following family owned prescriptions of herbal medicine in much higher. The reason for this, according to one commentator, is that "Chinese medicine is still an integral part of Taiwanese culture, despite the development of an advanced modern Western medical care system" (Chi 1994, 316). In the Province of British Columbia, Canada, there are in total over 200 practitioners of traditional Chinese medicine, with a similar number of retail outlets selling "packaged" traditional Chinese medications and herbs. The volume of the former category is about to CAD 8,000,000 per annum while the sale of herbs is reported to be worth another CAD 6,000,000 per annum. The enthusiasm for and usage of traditional Chinese medicine is also reflected by the increasing number of training schools for traditional Chinese medicine. A survey done in early 1998 shows that there are no less than twelve such schools providing training in this area of health care. This trend is probably also developing in other Chinese communities in Hong Kong, Singapore, New York, San Francisco, and Toronto.

Notes

1. The term "traditional Chinese medicine" can sometimes be misleading as if there is one homogeneous medical system practised by the Chinese people; this is not quite the case since the so-called Chinese people itself is made up of over 50 ethnic groups which over the last 2,000 years have contributed their own distinctive approaches to medicine due to ethnic, regional, and cultural differences. The more notable medical systems, named primarily after the names of their respective ethnic groups include "Han" medicine, Mongolian medicine, Tibetan medicine, Korean medicine, and so on. Since the "Han" ethnic group is the largest, Han medicine is predominant. The term "Chinese medicine" was adopted only in the nineteenth century after the importation of and for the purpose of differentiation from "Western medicine". The term "traditional Chinese medicine" has become popular after 1949 as an attempt to encourage and legitimize a more systematic and unified approach to an otherwise diversified group of medical practices.

2. The term *ch'i* has a variety of meanings and usages depending on the contexts; it is difficult, if not impossible, to use one English word to translate the term and to cover all its meanings.

3. For a brief discussion of the concept of "yin and yang" and the five phases/elements in the English language, consult Schwartz 1985, 350-382.

References

Chi, C. H. 1994. Integrating traditional medicine into modern health care systems: Examining the role of Chinese medicine in Taiwan. *Social Science & Medicine* 39, 3: 307-321.

Huang Ti. 1970. *Nei Ching Su Wen*. (The Yellow Emperor's classic of internal medicine) Ilza Veith (transl.), Berkeley: University of California Press.

Kleinman, A. et al. 1975. *Medicine in Chinese cultures*. U. S. Dept. of Health, Education and Welfare.

Lu, W. P. 1995. Chinese traditional medicine and the purpose of medicine. In *Medical goals. Life quality and medical ethics. Proceedings of the Eighth National Conference of Medical Ethics,* 117-119) China, Hunan, Zhang Jia Jie: The Medical Ethics Society of the Medical Association in China.

Schwartz, B. I. 1985. *The world of thought in ancient China*. Cambridge: BelKnap Press.

Su, W. J. et al. 1995. Report of questionnaire on the goals of medicine. In *Medical goals, Life quality and medical ethics. Proceedings of the Eighth National Conference of Medical Ethics,* 130-135) China, Hunan, Zhang Jia Jie: The Medical Ethics Society of the Medical Association in China.

Unschuld, P. U. 1985. *Medicine in China: A history of ideas*. Berkeley, London: University of California Press.

Chapter 4
Discourses on Health: A Critical Perspective

Joan Anderson and Sheryl Reimer Kirkham

We begin our inquiry into the discourses on health by recognizing that we too bring multiple perspectives and interpretations to the materials that we draw upon. As nurses and as academics, we share the "culture of health" (biomedicine as a culture itself) constructed from a "Western" classical liberal theory perspective. In this chapter we attempt to hold up to scrutiny, to reflect upon, and to question that which can easily be taken for granted as "the discipline", and the ring of "truth" that comes from the position of academic privilege.[1]

The critical perspective taken here is a consequence of conducting various research studies that have led us to examine what we mean by notions such as "culture" and "health". Anderson's research with women from racialized[2] groups who are living with a chronic illness led her to recognize the many layers of contexts in which people's experiences are enmeshed. Similarly, Reimer Kirkham's research with nurses revealed the complexity of intercultural encounters in health care settings. We came to understand culture not as a recipe for living (i.e. a static belief system) but rather as a complex, dynamic process grounded in everyday actions and enmeshed in the social and economic processes and relations of power between dominant and "subordinated" groups. The hegemonic practices of our own "culture of health" and the ways in which this culture has defined "problems" of the "other" became visible to us. We also came to understand that the ways in which we, as health professionals, speak about culture erases the structural inequities that organize people's experiences and lays the blame for their suffering on "their culture". Social problems become constructed as the problem of individuals and groups who subscribe to particular belief systems.

Through this journey of working with women, and through our own personal journeys and reflections on how we, as individuals, are situated and constructed, we have come to reframe our research through the lenses of a feminist, anti-racist, and post-colonial perspective. This perspective, we believe, gives us another way of understanding the concept of health. It also calls for a commitment to unmasking social injustices embedded within the relations of power between dominant and subordinated groups, that must intersect our discussion of health, illness, healing, and culture, if we are to move toward a discourse on ethics that is meaningful in the lives of those who have been marginalized and oppressed and who have often been constructed as the "cultural other".

Introduction

Woman with metastatic cancer: "I am really very healthy. I just have this problem but I am still me" (Kagawa-Singer 1993, 295)

What is it to be healthy? What is health? What is illness? The woman speaking, the sufferer, sees herself as healthy even though she is living with metastatic cancer, and may be seen as "diseased" from the perspective of Western biomedicine. Definitions of health and illness are multifarious and infused with personal, cultural, moral, religious, and social meanings. Jensen and Allen (1993) remind us that, "There are no universal norms of health; perceptions vary across individuals and cultures" (220). Discourses about health are fuelled not only by the theoretical and ideological perspectives that set disciplines and individuals apart from one another; differences within disciplines give rise to multiple ways of understanding and speaking about health, as is shown in Huch's 1991 paper that provides verbatim accounts of a panel discussion with six nursing leaders on the topic of health. Each participant's definition of health is derived from a particular "nursing theory" reflecting that knowledge is produced within different ideological frameworks and systems of meaning (Comaroff 1982; Lock and Gordon 1988) that can be found within a single discipline. What's more, people's definition of health may change over time; cultural meanings shift as one integrates new meanings and perspectives into one's stock of knowledge or as one grapples with a chronic or life threatening illness which demands a redefinition of self. One may come to see oneself as healthy even in the face of imminent death. In such instances health may embody spiritual and social meanings which were hitherto unknown.

Despite the lack of consensus about what health is, in the Western world at least, health is viewed, by individuals and governments alike, as a desirable state – as something "to be achieved". In Canada, for example, several government documents attest to this. *A new perspective on the health of Canadians* (Canada 1978) and *Achieving health for all: A framework for health promotion* (Canada 1986) were landmark policy documents that influenced government decision making about health and health care. In the United States, there was the national initiative for *Healthy People 2000* (Kulbok and Baldwin 1992; Public Health Service 1990) and the World Health Organisation (WHO) had a strategy for "Health for All" by the year 2000. The WHO (European Region) provided this definition of health in 1984:

> [Health is] [t]he extent to which an individual or group is able, on the one hand to develop aspirations and satisfy needs; and, on the other hand, to change or cope with the environment. Health is therefore seen as a resource for everyday life, not the objective of living; it is seen as a positive concept emphasizing social and personal resources, as well as physical capacities (British Columbia 1993a, 5).

So, far from being solely a personal matter, we are directed to consider the concept of health as having universal properties and as a state that should be aspired to by all. The WHO definition has been widely used by governments in directing health and social policy decisions. But this is only one definition of health; it is located within a paradigm that draws attention to the shift away from the "culture of biomedicine" to the broader sociopolitical and economic factors that shape the meaning and experiencing of health and illness. In the Western world, where biomedicine has been privileged, conceptions of health and illness have been enmeshed in systems of meanings that are distinctly biomedical. As Jones and Meleis (1993) suggest,

> The concept of health as an optimal disease-free state permeated both medicine and nursing for the first half of the 20th century until the World Health Organisation (WHO) proposed a definition of health as more than the absence of disease, focusing on the positive condition of physical, mental, and social well-being ... The WHO definition increased awareness of the complexity and multi-dimensionality of health and stimulated an inter-disciplinary debate (2).

Health as absence of disease; health as role performance; health as adaptation; health as maximizing human potential (Simmons 1989); these, and many more, make up the definitions of health from so-called "Western cultural perspectives". Changing definitions of health have been informed not only by the WHO but also by the critical examination of biomedicine. While conceptualizations from the social sciences have often been infused with biomedical meanings, a growing literature from the fields of "critical medical anthropology", the sociology of health, and the discipline of nursing offer a critique of the biomedical perspective, with its focus on the individualizing of health and ill health and the isolation of suffering from the social, economic, and political contexts (see, for example, Illich, Zola, McKnight, Caplan, and Shaiken 1977; Lock and Gordon 1988). Contemporary nursing scholars, in building a science of nursing that is distinct from biomedicine, have drawn upon critical and interpretative paradigms such as critical theory, phenomenology, and hermeneutics (see for example, Omery, Kasper, and Page 1995). Critiques have also come from a feminist perspective drawing attention to the intersectionality of gender, race,[3] and class in shaping definitions of health (see e.g. Anderson, Blue, and Lau 1993a; Anderson, Blue, Holbrook, and Ng 1993b; Bryan, Dadzie, and Scafe 1985; Oakley 1980; Omery, Kasper, and Page 1995; Sherwin 1992; Thompson, Allen, and Rodriques-Fisher 1992; Bolaria and Bolaria 1994). Perhaps definitions such as those from the WHO serve to legitimize perspectives that draw attention to the social context of health and illness.

We aim here not to add yet another definition of health; rather, we discuss different conceptualizations of health and the ideologies that underpin them, drawing upon the current literature as well as on our conversations with people from different ethnocultural communities. We examine, in particular, conceptualizations of health in relation to disease and extend this discussion to include the notions of health expressed by the people with whom we have spoken. Their notions, we believe, add a dimension that is not expressed in the literature. We then proceed to examine other conceptualizations of health that focus on health as personal responsibility. The counterpoint of this, we argue, are the contemporary discourses that focus on health as social responsibility and that emphasize the ways in which gender, race, and class relations structure the experience of health and well-being. We attend, in particular, to the ways in which feminist and post-colonial discourses are transforming conceptualizations of health and are thereby redefining ethical issues, as we shift our gaze from the paradigm of biomedicine to focus more sharply on the ways in which systemic injustice shapes the constructions of health within different populations. This chapter therefore draws attention to the multiple disciplinary and intellectual perspectives on health, illness, and disease that inform our understanding of cross-cultural health care ethics.

We are cognisant that what we have selected to address is framed from our own moral and ideological standpoints derived from feminist, anti-racist, and post-colonial discourses. Health and illness are not seen as concepts that are constructed from a neutral "cultural" perspective; rather, we want to show that conceptualizations of health and our experiencing of it are enmeshed in social, political, and economic contexts and underpinned by ideological meanings; what is claimed as "the culture" does not stand apart from these contexts but is inextricably interwoven into these systems of meaning.

Beyond binary conceptualizations of health and disease/illness: notions of holism

While there have been attempts to clarify the concepts of health, disease, and illness for the purposes of professional practice and research, in a review article, Jones and Meleis (1993) point to some of the confusion that still exists in stating precisely what we mean by health. Three conceptualizations in particular create confusion – health as a dichotomous variable, as a continuum, or as a more inclusive holistic state (2). An insightful perspective offered in the paper by Jones and Meleis is that the health–illness continuum is losing support and that a "health within illness" perspective is developing, whereby illness is seen as an event that can accelerate human growth (3).

Yet, despite attempts to construct definitions of health that are not refracted through the lenses of biomedicine, for the most part health still seems to be defined in relation to disease. In fact, Litva and Eyles (1994) suggest that as we examine different domains in which healing occurs – for example, the folk (non-medicalized specialized specialists), professional (biomedicine and professional healing traditions), and popular (home and community) – in every arena, health is seen in relation to disease. They proceed to point out that, "from a sociological view point, health is the absence of illness ... but as an absence of both disease and illness, health is seen negatively, as not being something" (1083). Saltonstall (1993) observes that, "[s]ociologists and anthropologists of medicine have largely focused their research on sickness and illness, thus obscuring social scientific investigations of health and healthiness" (7). So, a substantial literature glosses over what health is, while highlighting the distinctions between disease and illness. It appears that even when the concept of health is addressed, it receives only fleeting attention. Twaddle (1981), for example, seems to mention health as a way of introducing the notions of disease and illness. "Health" he suggests,

is increasingly being recognized as having psychological and social dimensions in addition to the biological ones. The term *"disease"* is used to indicate the biological dimension of non-health, which has come to be the focus of medicine in the past two centuries. Disease is an "objective" phenomenon that can be measured through laboratory tests, direct observation, or other "signs" ... *"Illness"* refers to the more subjective or psychological dimensions of non-health. (111-112)

Disease, as pathological abnormality, and illness, as the subjective experience of "ill health" (Field 1976; Idler 1979), are themes that run throughout the "medical" anthropology and sociology of health literature, and there is repeated reference to the distinctions between them. This shows the extent to which biomedical meanings infuse definitions of health even when there appears to be a flight from biomedicine to a perspective that is informed by the social science disciplines. Scheper-Hughes and Lock (1987) have remarked:

> As both medical anthropologists and clinicians struggle to view humans and the experience of illness and suffering from an integrated perspective, they often find themselves trapped by the Cartesian legacy. We lack a precise vocabulary with which to deal with mind-body-society interactions and so are left suspended in hyphens, testifying to the disconnectedness of our thoughts ...
>
> Ironically, the conscious attempts to temper the materialism and the reductionism of biomedical science often end up inadvertently recreating the mind/body opposition in a new form. For example, Leon Eisenberg (1977) elaborated the distinction between disease and illness ... While Eisenberg and his associates' paradigm has certainly helped to create a single language and discourse for both clinicians and social scientists, one unanticipated effect has been that physicians are claiming *both* aspects of the sickness experience for the medical domain. As a result, the "illness" dimension of human distress (i.e. the social relations of sickness) are being medicalized and individualized, rather than politicized and collectivized. Medicalization inevitably entails a missed identification between the individual and the social bodies, and a tendency to transform the social into the biological. (10)

While Scheper-Hughes and Lock see physicians as claiming both aspects of the "sickness" experience, Twaddle (1982) draws our attention to the implications that the fracturing of disease and illness into separate entities has for the professional division of labour. Nursing is claiming, he suggests,

> that the care, as opposed to cure, of the patient with central attention to illness (the subjective, psychological component of poor health) and sickness (the social component) ... is their central focus. Medicine, according to this ideology, can be left to diagnosis and treatment of disease, nursing can take over the care of sick people. (341)

That nursing would see illness management as within its domain does not minimize the concerns raised by Scheper-Hughes and Lock; if indeed "illness" is "the social relations of sickness" then the social is being transformed into an arena for professional management. It could well be argued that the carving up of "disease" and "illness" between different professional groups reifies human suffering and extends professional hegemony over the lives of ordinary people. Current discourses on health that construct it as within the purview of the practice of health professionals may also carry the potential for further extension of professional control into everyday life.

Central to the works cited here is the idea of health in opposition to disease and illness, and disease and illness as distinct from one another. Disease and illness emerge as two distinct entities – one biomedical, the other socially constructed. Health is understood by their absence, or in conceptual opposition to both. The understanding of illness as socially constructed may be extended to acknowledge that certain diseases can be similarly understood. Scholars such as Sherwin (1992) and Singer and Baer (1995) point out how certain practices and experiences have been medicalized to become diseases within the Western context. Singer and Baer present the example of homosexuality: "Efforts to pathologize homo-sexuality have been tied to a larger social attempt to control the behaviour of gay men and lesbians" (80). Ultimately, pressure from the gay community resulted in the deletion of homosexuality from the psychiatric nomenclature of the Diagnostic and Statistical Manual. Similarly, the experiences of menstruation have been medicalized as premenstrual syndrome (PMS). Thus, in our efforts to elucidate illness and disease we are reminded of the extent to which both illness and disease are, in fact, socially constructed.

The binary conceptualization of health in relation to illness and disease carries implications beyond the oversight described above. Health through its association with disease and illness is limited to a predominantly physical realm and is therefore primarily biologically defined. Gordon's (1988) explication of the assumptions underpinning Western medicine is helpful in uncovering the degree to which biomedicine influences understandings of health. She points out that as a product of Western culture and society, biomedicine draws on dominant Western philosophical traditions such as naturalism and individualism. The commitment to a physicalist view of health and illness is influenced by the naturalist assertions regarding the autonomy of "nature" from human consciousness, culture, society, and time and space. The Cartesian dualism of mind and body is implicated in the naturalist stance, as are a materialist commitment and a rationalist epistemology.

Reality is directly proportional to materiality, which is considered lacking in

spirit; the more physical, the more real. "Body" is distinct from "mind" ...
Health and illness are defined in terms of materialist indicators, such as blood
pressure, rather than "spirit", such as "feeling" healthy. (Gordon 1988, 24)

A conceptualization of health as holistic stands in contrast to this binary,
physicalist view of health. While the holistic health movement has only
recently been gaining momentum in North America it has a long-standing
history within "non-Western" communities.[4] Conversations with people,
some of whom seldom have their voices included in the "academic"
discourse on health, give another perspective on health. Some of these
perspectives follow.

Women and men speak of health: The notion of holism

In our efforts to include the voices of experts from Vancouver communities,
we have had several long conversations with eight people, six of whom were
of non-European heritage, and who felt entitled to speak about the
constructions of health from different cultural perspectives, including the
biomedical perspective.[5] These conversations provided an opportunity to
enrich our conceptualizations derived from the "academic" literature, and
opened up new ways of thinking about health. While the constructions of
health varied among the people with whom we have spoken, one thing stood
out. Health was generally viewed as "holistic" – this is not to say that the
word held similar meanings for everyone, yet for the majority, health
encompassed different dimensions of life. For example, one participant from
the Indo-Canadian community, made the following point:

> The word "sehat" is more or less the exact translation of the word "health",
> but the word "sehat" means the well-being of the entire individual.
> Obviously, the word "sehat" does not distinguish between physical health
> and mental health, and neither does the word health. It is our practice in the
> biomedical model to distinguish between such aspects and in practice that is
> very evident ... "Holistic" health is not a word used in other cultures
> because the words "sehat" covers that idea.

Josephine (Pseudonym) had this to say about health:

> I guess the way I would define health is the overall well-being of an
> individual – physical, mental, and emotional. And it's interesting because I
> would assume that the broader definition of health would be one certainly the
> aboriginal communities of the Americas would support and buy into ... Both
> people of European ancestry and people of Colour and Aboriginal people
> who have a close connection to their cultural roots see a broader meaning of
> health rather than the narrow ... I think the definition is shared with people
> from a variety of cultural backgrounds ... I think that certainly for those of us
> from diverse communities that have been educated to a certain level in a
> particular model – in a particular way – our sense is that we have adopted a

different approach to a certain extent to health and we've had to pull or re-learn some of our original perceptions of what good health was.

This person goes on to weave the discussion of health into health care:

And if you have an ulcer, it may mean there is a particular medical cause ... And I think that historically though, what needs to happen is people would not only look at the causal effect but look at the whole environment to see what else was going on for that individual, and taking a much more holistic approach to what might be the cause, and how not only that individual but the family and community around the individual might support the individual to get help, and see that the ulcer is only one causal effect of other things going on in the person's life.

This is another participant's perspective on what health means:

I look at health in a very holistic way. It's my Chinese background that does that to me. The way you live, what you eat, physically how you look after yourself, clothing you wear. The Chinese really think of it – hot and cold foods depending on how you are feeling. I just come with that kind of natural orientation, so health to me has to do with mental health and social relationships as well, so it's a whole life-style ...

To me if you are ill or have a disease or whatever, there's something about your life-style, there's blockage there. Of course, it could be genetic too, I suppose you could be born with some sort of problem. My concept is really that life is a matter of balance, and getting the right balance in terms of food, in terms of life-style, in terms of relationships, in terms of emotions. When you are ill it means something is really not working the way it should. One has to take corrective measures to get that balance right.

What has been striking as we have reviewed our conversations with the men and women who agreed to speak with us, is the extent to which their notions of holism seem to differ from notions that underpin "Western" inter-pretations of holistic health. For example, "holism" has now been couched in the language of health promotion and middle class constructions of the healthy body. Lupton (1995) observes the growing discourse around holistic health.

Good health has become a visible sign, demonstrated by the lean, taut, exercising body. The holistic model expands the definition of health to include feelings of self-empowerment and autonomy, a potential for self-improvement, and spiritual equilibrium. Such a philosophy of health, encompassing all dimensions of a person's life, is evident in the literature of alternative therapies but is also pervasive in health promotional discourses. (71)

This popularized perspective on holistic health has come under critical scru-tiny by some of the people with whom we spoke. As one participant put it,

This New Age movement in health in North America, most of it I find is really off the wall ... Some of the people who are making millions of dollars talking about other cultures, religions, remedies, and practices don't know a darn thing about what they are talking about because they have never studied these cultures or traditions. What they are presenting is pop culture of New Age, not what the reality in the ancient healing and medical system is ... I think they are doing a disservice to the origins of old systems of health. The reason they are able to get away with spouting such uninformed material is because nobody is questioning them ... Without knowing what it really is, just saying "vegetarianism is good", without recognizing how vegetarianism was practised under yoga when the tradition was developed or the way that tradition evolved.

The biomedical model itself has never said that anything except the biomedical model is worthwhile. In the old cultures that have developed over thousands of years, people have been treating illness for thousands of years, so there is some good that exists there.

We turn now to other perspectives on health, that have gained considerable ground in North America. We start by examining one perspective, which like the biomedical perspective is rooted in the ideology of individualism and proceed to other constructions that view health as social responsibility.

Beyond personal responsibility:
Collective experiences and social responsibility for health

Achieving health/wellness through personal responsibility:
the moral imperative

In a book published in 1990, *The seeds of health: Promoting wellness in the 1990s*, a paper by Sister Roberta Freeman starts by reminding us of the excellent health care system in Canada, of which we should be justifiably proud, and the price we must pay for it. She goes on to say:

However, the morbidity and mortality rates we experience in our country, in spite of the various means which are readily available to prevent illness, should be of greater concern. These include a varied and abundant food supply, a safe water supply, the wherewithal for universal immunization programs and an economic situation whereby, under normal circumstances, a balance of work and leisure are distinct possibilities for most people ... I put forward the proposition that for health preservation and promotion to be achieved, it is essential that individuals become inculcated with a deep sense of personal responsibility for their own health and that of others. (1, 2)

The paper captures, we think, the individualist ideology that is at the core of the health promotion/wellness movement, with its message to adopt healthy – or healthier – life-styles; individual efforts are responsible for success, and "every person is the architect of his or her own fortune, since equal opportunity is available to everyone" (Li 1988, 5). The belief that health is "a good to be pursued" and that it is a personal responsibility (with the implicit notion of "good citizen") puts health within the grasp of all, if only we put our minds to it. This is tied to a definition of health as self-actualizing and health as a holistic realization of one's potential (Freeman 1990). As Sister Freeman puts it, "If one's physical, mental, social and spiritual needs have been met, then wholeness of being and the experience of health as defined by the World Health Organisation should be the reality" (6).

An analysis of the health and wellness movement by Peter Conrad (1994) provides important insights into positions like the one taken by Sister Freeman. His analysis begins to unmask the *raison d'être* of the wellness /health promotion movement, and perhaps helps us to see the conception of "personal responsibility" not as a punitive jab at the underclass (deprived as they are of material resources and the wherewithal to purchase what is needed – for example, adequate food and shelter – to promote health), but rather as tied to deeper moral issues within Western society. Health activities, Conrad (1994) points out, can be seen as a form of cultural regeneration at a time of social debility. "A metaphysical line was forged between health and the vitality of the nation. Physical development was seen as recharging vitality, and perhaps more importantly, a step toward human perfection" (386). He goes on to tell us that "[m]orality and health are often linked", and our usage of terms like a sick society, a healthy society, point to the moral valence that these words have (387). "In short", Conrad argues, "health and health-promotion behaviours are frequently depicted as the good while disease and putatively disease-producing behaviours are seen as bad" (388). Referring to Gillick (1984) he notes:

> She argues that in a society as morally ambiguous as ours there are few commonly accepted ways of individual moral action. The pursuit of fitness and wellness has become a path of individual and moral action. To pursue health and fitness for yourself and society are unambiguous goods. The pursuit of wellness becomes the pursuit of the good life …the good life has become the healthy life. (388-9)

The pursuit of health seems to provide hope that our individual actions can collectively regenerate and make "wholesome" what has come to be seen as a "sick" society.

While Conrad's paper offers important insights, it poses questions. There is little doubt that there are layers of moral meanings in the health promotion/wellness movement. Yet, it is not entirely clear that governments are intent on promoting health and wellness solely for the purpose of strengthening the moral fibre of the nation. While the message from governments and the advocates of the health promotion/ wellness movement might be couched in terms to appeal to our moral sensibilities, could it be that cost containment might be the real incentive for health promotion?

It should not escape our attention that several different and sometimes conflicting messages are embedded in documents such as *Achieving health for all: A framework for health promotion* (Canada 1986). On the one hand the barriers to health are recognized. On the other hand, self-care and personal and community responsibility are emphasized. While on the surface these appear as meritorious and reasonable expectations of "good citizenship", they nonetheless pave the way for rationalizing off-loading the responsibility for health and health care to individuals and their families. The message about responsibility for self is not only about taking responsibility to be healthy and to stay healthy; it's also about taking responsibility for health care.

The ideology of personal responsibility that infuses the domains of health and health care carries a set of expectations that may not be immediately apparent. Scholars who critique this ideology point out that there may be negative consequences on the health of families, in particular, on the health of women who, for a variety of reasons, usually take on the lion's share of the care giving role. Angus (1994) argues, "The women who shoulder the burden of cost containment in health care ... face a legacy of poverty or lost income, as well as immediate restrictions to personal time and space" (36). Giving up employment to take on the care of an ill family member translates into loss of income and loss of pension, which might mean a life of poverty in old age; 47.4 percent of single women over the age of 65 live in poverty (British Columbia 1994). This number might increase as more women leave the paid workforce to assume unpaid care giving roles.

As the Western physicalist views of health, influenced by biomedicine, are in contrast to the holistic perspectives described by the people with whom we have spoken, so also is the individual experience of health as furthered by the health promotion movement in contrast to a more collective view of health. Gordon (1988), in her discussion of naturalism and individualism as two "tenacious" assumptions in Western medicine, suggests that the person in Western tradition is distinguished from his/her social position, role, and culture to the extent that "[t]he individual has distinct priority in the individual/society equation" (34). The view that health belongs to the individual is in keeping with this individualistic "I-self" ideology. However, those who hold to a more collective "we-self" view understand health as enmeshed in the context and contingencies of everyday life – the environment, the family, and the community. This was reflected in the perspective of one of the people with whom we spoke who was constructing the notion of health as he perceived it within the Chinese culture:

> Health has family and social aspects for every individual within the Chinese cultural context. When we were young, we were taught that you have to take care of your body, because when you take care of your body you are doing good for your parents ... When we were young, every time our parents asked us to put on lots of clothes when we went out, they would say, "take care of your body and you will do good to your parents and you will be a good kid."
>
> In this aspect, the motivation to keep oneself healthy is a family obligation ... Another aspect to being healthy is the informal care among the family. The family has 100% obligation to care for other members in certain kinds of illness or trouble ... so we have a very heavy sense that we have to take care of our family members if someone gets sick.

Some of the people with whom we spoke were convinced that health could not be understood outside of the context of family relationships. Furthermore, they felt that women played a key role in defining and maintaining health in their families; the health needs of their family, as they perceived them, often took priority over their own, as reflected in this woman's statement:

> I'm not sure that most women when they think of their own health, their well-being in terms of their being healthy, that they only think of the context of them, themselves. They see it as their well-being is connected, not dependent on, but connected to the well-being of other people that they care about. And I don't think most men see it that way ...
>
> It was really interesting, I have been at the last hours at a number of friends and all of them have talked about looking after their partners, all the women have. And I think that is something particularly female in my experience.

We suggest that these constructions of health are grounded in a complex nexus of social, cultural, political, and economic meanings. They alert us to the differential constructions that can arise within particular cultural contexts; for example, the notion of balance within the Chinese culture. We also get a glimpse into the gendering of health. These differing constructions inform us of the multiple ways in which holistic health is understood and interpreted.

Reframing the definitions:
Determinants of health and illness – health as social responsibility

> [Health] is seen as a positive concept emphasizing social and personal resources, as well as physical capacities (WHO, cited in British Columbia 1993a, 5)

In the last decade the discourse on health has taken a new turn. Biomedical definitions and individualistic notions are giving way to social meanings and definitions, and we are asked not only to define what health is, but what makes it accessible, as a resource for living, to some and not to others. Robert Evans (1994a), in the opening paragraph of the Introduction to the book, *Why are some people healthy and others not?,* captures the central point in the discussion about health and its determinants:

> Top people live longer. Moreover they are generally healthier while doing so. This is not exactly news. Many studies, in many countries, over many years, have shown a correlation between life expectancy and various measures of social status – income, education, occupation, residence ... Studies of the living, while fewer because decent health information is so scarce ... show that health status is also correlated with social status. And such studies confirm what most people knew anyway – poverty is bad for you. As Sophie Tucker said, "I've been poor, and I've been rich. Rich is better." (3)

Evans goes on, of course, to tell us that it is not as simple as it looks. Rich is better – but there are other things as well! Why some people are healthy and others not, is complex. Marmot's well-known Whitehall study, cited by Evans, was carried out with more than ten thousand civil servants over nearly two decades. In none of the groups were people impoverished – all were employed and reasonably well paid compared to the general population. Even among this relatively homogeneous group there was a gradient in mortality from the top to bottom of the hierarchy, with mortality increasing as one went down the scale. Evans suggests that the main point of Marmot's findings is that there is something that powerfully influences health, and that is correlated with hierarchy (Evans 1994, 5-7).

The information that would help us to understand why some people are healthy and others not, is far from complete. Yet, review of mortality rates by social class (Black Report, cited by Evans) shows higher mortality rates in the lower social classes persisting since the data were first collected in 1911, even though the causes of death have changed radically during that period (Evans 1994, 8-11). All these findings have led Evans to conclude that there is extensive evidence for correlation between health and hierarchical position within populations, and that the connections between health and social environment are very real and may be very powerful (Evans 1994b). These determinants, of course, have nothing to do with health care. Evans therefore makes the case that if an overdeveloped health care system drains away resources that might have been used to improve the social environment, then this could be seen as a threat to health (4).

Evans is not alone in highlighting the social determinants of health. Government documents, such as *A new perspective on the health of*

Canadians (Canada 1978) and *Achieving health for all: A framework for health promotion* (Canada 1986), have all acknowledged these determinants, along with documents such as *New directions for a healthy British Columbia* (British Columbia 1993), and *The Moderator's report from the Women's Health Conference* (British Columbia 1993b). We quote from this report:

> Women and men suffer the repercussions of the social determinants of health: the inequities of our society that make a person more susceptible to illness and disease. Studies have shown that the determinants of health include such wide-ranging factors as income, stress, empowerment, personal-support networks, marital status, education and housing. (6-7)

Other scholars have pointed to the stressors of everyday life that influence the health of certain groups, and Jones and Meleis (1993) argue that primary stressors may originate in social factors such as ethnicity and gender in addition to social class. They suggest that resources may enable people to manage stressors, and that the extent to which personal and social resources – e.g. social support, and economic resources – are available plays a decisive role in managing health (6). "Availability of these resources", they argue, "varies widely, partly because social systems embody unequal distribution of resources, and is partly related to the extent that personal and social resources are mobilized" (Jones and Meleis 1993, 7). They suggest that it's not only a matter of resources being available; people must also be able to utilize the resources, hence their focus on empowerment, which they argue is enabling (8).

The discourse on the "determinants" of health has not escaped critical scrutiny. Hayes (1994), while acknowledging the contributions to our understandings of relationships in human health that the determinants of health perspective have offered, draws attention to some points of tension. He notes that although there is recognition of the complexity of relationships influencing population health, different dimensions such as the social environment, physical environment, and biological endowment are not theorized together "as mutually constitutive, coexisting dimensions of being" (124). Dimensions are presented sequentially, whereas in reality, he points out, individuals are influenced simultaneously by such factors and presumably by others. Hayes suggests that the simultaneity of influences upon human health and the interactive ways in which multiple co-existing influences might operate are not addressed by looking at health determinants in a sequential way (125). This will require "consideration of the spatiality of lived experience, to understand the (potentially) multitudinous ways in which salient dimensions of influence get played out across and through space-time in the lives of individuals" (127).

The need to recognize that factors operate simultaneously in the lives of individuals is underscored by Black feminist intellectuals such as Rose Brewer (1993). She has argued that the "polyvocality of multiple social locations is historically missing from … mainstream academic disciplines" (13). Running through Black feminist analysis is the principle of the simultaneity of oppression, which calls for a rethinking of the social structure of inequality in the context of race, class, and gender intersections (16). A growing body of literature by post-colonial and feminist scholars is illuminating how the simultaneity of gender, race, and class oppression shapes experiences of health and well-being (see, for example, Ahmad 1993; Bolaria 1988; Bryan, Dadzie, and Scafe 1985; Lock 1990; Muszynski 1994; Roberts 1992). Bryan, Dadzie, and Scafe, who conceptualize health as encompassing the physical, mental, and social dimensions, discuss the ways in which our "working conditions, the standard of our housing, our access to health and welfare services and the treatment we receive from them" (91) influence our health. Black women in Britain, they argue, have tolerated the lowest paid jobs and least satisfactory working conditions; the social and economic conditions outside of their control have shaped their experiences of health. These scholars, among others, have drawn attention to the social injustices and systemic inequities that determine how health is experienced by people of Colour living in industrialized nations; racism, sexism, and systemic discrimination and injustice undermine life opportunities and are barriers to health and well-being. There is the call to focus not only on the inter-connections among gender inequality, racialization, and health, but also on how inequities might be addressed.

The ways in which life context shapes the experiencing of health was profoundly understood by the people with whom we have spoken, some of whom, through the process of uprooting and resettling, had first-hand experience with social and economic inequities. Others have worked in situations where the realities of everyday life and the effects of poverty were starkly visible in the lives of people who sought assistance from health and social service providers. The following account reflects the awareness of the people with whom we spoke of the multiple forces that intersect to influence health:

> there are significant other issues that affect one's sense of well-being. And certainly, I guess Trevor Hancock, a physician who's been working for a number of years recently said it best of all, "It's difficult to feel if you are starving or you are cold in the rain." … I think one of the interesting issues in this country in particular, is that technology and the infrastructure that are built up around the so-called health care system – it has little to do with health, and everything to do with acute medical care and nothing else.

Concluding comments

The preceding discussion shows that health can be discussed in various ways, and that the concept is infused with multiple meanings even within the health professions. Contemporary discourses, such as those derived from a feminist, post-colonial perspective, direct us not to see health from a neutral standpoint of belief systems stripped of social context. Understanding the meaning of health within the context of culture requires a conceptualization of culture as a complex network of meanings enmeshed within historical, social, economic, and political processes. The discourse on health must of necessity explicate the intersectionality and simultaneity of race, gender, and class relations, the practice of racialization, the connectedness to historical context, and how the curtailment of life opportunities created by structural inequities influences health.

In Canada, where Multiculturalism is official government policy, and where health care providers are encouraged to be "culturally sensitive", the meaning of health is often seen as located within particular cultural contexts. Culture here takes on the quality of a "thing" possessed by some groups (the so called "mainstream" escapes the gaze) and becomes the explanatory framework for understanding health and illness behaviours of those constructed as "other" – "cultural minorities". This is not a neutral position, but has consequences for the lives of those constructed as the "cultural other". Human misery and suffering can be neatly explained in terms of belief systems; the many layers of contexts in which individual experiences are embedded, and the complex interweaving of cultural meanings, economic relations, and relations of power and domination can be glossed over or denied.

A central issue in this chapter is that theorizing about health and culture is not a benign scholarly activity, but has consequences for the theories we construct about cross-cultural health care ethics and practical implications for people's lives. Viewing health as a responsibility of the individual, or as located within static belief systems – "the culture" – will lead us in an entirely different direction than locating health within a web of social and political relationships. If we believe, for example, that the simultaneity of different forms of oppression located in history structure life opportunities and that this has major implications for people's health, then we will call for the unmasking of the social injustices located in histories of colonization, oppression, dehumanization, and depersonalization, wherever they may exist. Any consideration of ethical issues will need to take into account the multilayered contexts in which human experiences are situated. In particular, there must be attention to the power differential that operates insidiously as dominant groups "represent" the situation of subordinated groups. If we recognize the complex relations of ruling and domination, then we will need to envision an ethics of health care that extends beyond issues of individual rights to include the larger issue of social justice for groups that have historically been racialized, marginalized, and oppressed.

An issue that is being raised in the discussions about health, and which was poignantly addressed by one of the people with whom we spoke in doing the research for this chapter, is that the allocation of added resources for health care may not translate into better health for the population; indeed the reverse might be true. So the issue is not just the allocation of resources within health care, but rather, the allocation of resources between health care *and* health – for example, the pressing need to address poverty, which is connected to racism and sexism and exploitation of the underclass. How will decisions be made about resource allocation and about addressing social inequities and issues of racism, sexism, and poverty? What ethical issues might be anticipated? What role will health care ethics play? And what will all this mean for the construction of theories of cross-cultural health care ethics? The dialogue is just beginning. Addressing such questions will be the challenge of the future.

Notes

1. We thank Peter Stephenson for his insightful comments during the initial review of the ideas for this paper which prompted us to consider the ways in which the WHO definition of health legitimates concerns about health determinants.

2. We use the term racialization here as it is used by Cashmore, quoted in Ahmad (1993): "[racialization] refers to a political and ideological process by which particular populations are identified by direct or indirect reference to their real or imagined phenotypical characteristics in such a way as to suggest that the population can only be understood as supposedly biological entity" (18).

3. We use the term race, not as a biological entity, but as a socially constructed category, and as it is defined by Higginbotham, quoted by Brewer (1993), "[R]ace must be seen as a social construction predicated upon the recognition of difference and signifying the simultaneous distinguishing and positioning of groups vis-à-vis one another. More than this, race is a highly contested representation of relations of power between social categories by which individuals are identified and identify themselves" (16-17).

4. We draw upon Aihwa Ong's (1988) definition of Western. "'Western' is taken here to include European societies under prewar British and postwar American hegemonic leadership" (90).

5. We are indebted to the people who participated in these conversations. We have received permission from some of these people to acknowledge them by either name or organization. Others did not give their permission to have their own names or the names of their organizations included so they are not mentioned here. Beverly Nann; Sadie Kuehn; United Chinese Community Enrichment Services Society (S.U.C.C.E.S.S.); Ruth Coles, Dianne Doyle, Providence Health Care, Mount Saint Joseph's Hospital; Shashi Assanand, Vancouver and Lower Mainland Multicultural Family Support Services; Guninder C.

Mumick, Multicultural Health Education Consultant, Vancouver/Richmond Health Board.

References

Ahmad, W. (Ed.). 1993. *"Race" and health in contemporary Britain.* Buckingham, England: Open University Press.

Anderson, James. 1983. Health and illness in Pilipino immigrants. Cross-cultural medicine. *Western Journal of Medicine* 139: 811-819.

Anderson, J., C. Blue, and A. Lau. 1993a. Women's perspectives on chronic illness: ethnicity, ideology and restructuring of life. *Social Science and Medicine* 33 (2), 101-113.

Anderson, J., C. Blue, A. Holbrook, and M. Ng. 1993b. On chronic illness: Immigrant women in Canada's work force: A feminist perspective. *Canadian Journal of Nursing Research* 25 (2),7-22.

Angus, J. 1994. Women's paid/unpaid work and health: Exploring the social context of everyday life. *The Canadian Journal of Nursing Research* 26 (4), 23-42.

Bolaria, B. S. 1988. The health effects of powerlessness: Women and racial minority immigrant workers. In *Sociology of health care in Canada,* ed. B. S. Bolaria and H. D. Dickenson, 439-459. Toronto: Harcourt, Brace, Jovanovich.

Bolaria, B. S. and R. Bolaria, R. 1994. *Women, Medicine and Health.* Halifax: Fernwood Publishing.

Brewer, R. M. 1993. Theorizing race, class and gender: The new scholarship of Black feminist intellectuals and Black women's labour. In *Theorizing Black feminisms: The visionary pragmatism of Black women,* ed. S. M. James, and A. P. A. Busia, 13-30. London: Routledge.

Bryan, B., S. Dadzie, and S. Scafe. 1985. *The heart of the race: Black women's lives in Britain.* London: Virgo Press

British Columbia. 1993a. New Directions for a healthy British Columbia. Province of British Columbia: Ministry of Health and Ministry Responsible for Seniors.

British Columbia. 1993b. Women's Health Conference: Moderator's Report. B.C.: Ministry of Health and Ministry Responsible for Seniors.

British Columbia. 1994. A Report on the health of British Columbians: Provincial Health Officer's Annual Report. B.C.: Ministry of Health and Ministry Responsible for Seniors.

Canada. 1978. A new perspective on the health of Canadians: A working document. Ottawa: Minister of Supply and Services.

Canada. 1986. Achieving health for all: A framework for health promotion. Ottawa: Minister of Supply and Services.

Comaroff, J. 1982. Medicine: Symbol and ideology. In *The problem of medical knowledge: Examining the social construction of medicine,* ed. P. Wright and A. Treacher, 49-68. Edinburgh: Edinburgh University Press.

Conrad, P. 1994. Wellness as virtue: Morality and the pursuit of health. *Culture, Medicine and Psychiatry* (18), 385-401.

Evans, R. 1994a. Introduction. In *Why are some people healthy and others not? The determinants of health of populations,* ed. R. Evans, M. Barer, and T. Marmor, 3-26. New York: Aldine De Gruyter.

Evans, R. 1994b. Health care as a threat to health: Defense, opulence, and the social environment. *Daedalus: Journal of the American Academy of Arts and Sciences* 123 (4), 21-42.

Field, D. 1976. The social definition of illness. In *An introduction to medical sociology*, ed. D. Tuckett, 334-366. London: Tavistock Publications.

Freeman, Sister Roberta. 1990. Health: A personal responsibility. In *The seeds of health: Promoting wellness in the 1990's*, ed. G. Eikenberry, 1-8. Ottawa: The Canadian College of Health Service Executives.

Gordon, D. 1988. Tenacious assumptions in Western medicine. In *Biomedicine examined*, ed. M. Lock and D. Gordon, 19-56. Dordrecht, Holland: Kluwer Academic Publishers.

Hayes, M. 1994. Evidence, determinants of health and population epidemiolgy: Humming the tune, learning the lyrics. In *The determinants of population health: A critical assessment*, ed. M. Hayes, L. Foster, and H. Foster, 121-133. Western Geographical Series, Vol. 29, University of Victoria.

Huch, M. H. 1991. Perspectives on health. *Nursing Science Quarterly* 4 (1), 33-40.

Idler, E. L. (1979). Definitions of health and illness and medical sociology. *Social Science and Medicine* 13A, 723-731.

Illich, I., I. K. Zola, J. McKnight, J. Caplan, and H. Shaiken. 1977. *Disabling professions*. New York: Maryon Boyars.

Jensen, l. M. and Allen. 1993. Wellness: The dialectic of illness. *Image: Journal of Nursing Scholarship* 25 (3), 220-224.

Jones, P. and A. I. Meleis. 1993. Health is empowerment. *Advances in Nursing Science* 15 (3), 1-14.

Kagawa-Singer, M. 1993. Re-defining health: Living with cancer. *Social Science and Medicine* 37 (3), 295-304.

Kulbok, P. A. and J. H. Baldwin. 1992. From preventive health behavior to health promotion: Advancing a positive construct of health. *Advances in Nursing Science* 14 (4), 50-64.

Li, P. 1988. *Ethnic inequality in a class society*. Toronto: Thompson Educational Publishing, Inc.

Litva, A., and J. Eyles. 1994. Health or healthy: Why people are not sick in a Southern Ontarian town. *Social Sciences and Medicine* 39 (8),1083-1091.

Lock, M. 1990. On being ethnic: The politics of identity breaking and making in Canada, or nerva on Sunday. *Culture, Medicine and Psychiatry* 14, 237-254.

Lock, M. and D. Gordon (Eds.). 1988. *Biomedicine examined*. Dordrecht: Kluwer Academic Press.

Lupton, D. 1995. *The imperative of health: Public health and the regulated body*. London, England: Sage Publications.

Muszynski, A. 1994. Gender inequality and life chances: Women's lives and health. In *Women , Medicine and Health*, ed. B. Bolaria and R. Bolaria, 57-72). Halifax, NS: Fernwood Publishing.

Oakley, A. 1980. *Women confined: Towards a sociology of childbirth*. Oxford: Martin Robinson.

Omery, A.,C. E. Kasper, and G. G. Page. 1995. *In search of nursing science*. Thousand Oaks: Sage.

Ong, Aihwa. 1988. Colonialism and modernity: Feminist re-presentations of women in non-Western societies. *Inscriptions* 3/4, 79-93.

Public Health Service. 1990. *Healthy people 2000: National health promotion and disease prevention objectives*. Conference Edition. Summary. Washington, DC: U.S. Government Printing Office.

Roberts, H. (Ed.). 1992 *Women's health matters*. London: Routledge.

Saltonstall, R. 1993. Healthy bodies, social bodies: Men's and women's concepts and practices of health in everyday life. *Social Sciences and Medicine* 36 (1), 7-14.

Scheper-Hughes, N. and M. Lock. 1987. The mindful body: A prolegomenon to future work in medical anthropology. *Medical Anthropology Quarterly* 1(1), 6-41.

Sherwin, S. 1992. *No longer patient: Feminist ethics and health care.* Philadelphia: Temple University Press.

Simmons, S. J. 1989. Health: A concept analysis. *International Journal of Nursing Studies* 26 (2), 155-161.

Singer, M., and H. Baer. 1995. *Critical medical anthropology.* Amityville, New York: Baywood Publishing.

Thompson, J. L., D. Allen, and L. Rodriques-Fisher (Eds.). 1992. *Critique, resistance and action: Working papers in the politics of nursing.* New York: National League for Nursing.

Twaddle, A. 1982. From medical sociology to the sociology of health: Some changing concerns in the sociological study of sickness and treatment. In *Sociology the state of the art,* ed. T. Bottomore, S. Nowak, and M. Sokolowska, 323-358. London: Sage Publications.

Twaddle, A. 1981. Sickness and the sickness career: Some implications. In *The relevance of social science for medicine,* ed. L. Eisenberg and A. Kleinman, 112-133. Dordrecht: D. Reidel Publishing Co.

Chapter 5
Expanding Notions of Culture
for Cross-Cultural Ethics in Health and Medicine

Peter Stephenson

Par le même acte, grâce auquel il tisse la langue hors de lui, [l'homme] s'y tisse lui-même (Von Humbolt, cited in Cassirer 1973, 18)

Man is an animal suspended in webs of significance he himself has spun. (Geertz 1973, 5)

It has recently become regarded as useful by persons doing "health promotion" to include "culture" among a cluster of variables to be taken into account in the decisions people make when they become ill. Likewise, the term culture has found its way into the manifold clinical concerns of medical ethicists, health administrators, nurses, and physicians. Because many different assumptions lie behind various uses of the term culture, it is important for researchers and practitioners to be aware of these. For some writers culture is shared learned behaviour; for others it is a patterned abstraction from behaviour. Some researchers think culture exists in the mind (as ideational) while others see it as consisting of observable things and events in the external world (as material).

This chapter focuses on examples that are meant to both illustrate and clarify some problematic uses of the culture concept as opposed to taking a position on any particular definition.[1] We may begin somewhat reflexively by noting that an operationalized view of culture as simply one intervening variable among many is actually the hallmark of a particular culture which tends to see everything in instrumental terms. In other words, the view that culture is a relatively insignificant determinant of human behaviour is itself a core cultural belief – particularly in Western economics, science, and medicine. I contend in this chapter that an essentially trivial notion of culture has played havoc with the construction of ethics by greatly constraining the range of issues that are regarded as part of the discourse on ethics.

Expanding our understanding of culture to include the wider contexts within which all people operate during communication in culturally plural situations means yielding a privileged position for the authoritative professional whose views are no less cultural than those of her clients. Appreciating how culture obscures as well as reveals certain connections to people in various contexts related to healing and illness is the goal of our understanding. However culture might be defined, as a universal feature of human social life it must apply equally to those who provide services and those who receive them. In the field of health and illness this means that how clinicians create meaning when interacting with their clientele interests us at least as much as the illness experiences of their clients. Most importantly, it is the dominant culture (that of the researchers, physicians, ethicists, anthropologists, etc.) which may be especially difficult to analyse and comprehend. This is particularly the case for medical practice and research because there it is often assumed that such a quintessential realm of science and logic has become a privileged site where culture (in its ideological and subjective sense) does not play a role – that biomedicine is neutral or culture-free. Or, if it does play a role, culture is simply viewed as a contaminating variable to be excluded from analysis or included in a controlled manner.

In this chapter it is suggested that regarding culture as a minor and contaminating variable is actually basic to how the most central ideological construct of industrial Western culture is reproduced; that is, by asserting that it is not an ideology in the first place. Much of medical science manifests an unwavering belief (an ideology) in which it is maintained that it is not itself an ideology, but that it constitutes the truth revealed through experimental methods. Culture is seen as a controlled factor in experimental modalities. The experimental method is not recognized as a cultural form where certain ideas are reproduced, especially the notion that means are justified by ends. If a cross-cultural ethics is to ever develop in pluralist societies, such privileged and hegemonic orientations will have to be subverted through an expanded self-awareness on the part of practitioners and researchers. Modern medical science will have to recognize that it itself is a culture. The realm of ethics – concerned as it ultimately must be with both the examination and creation of alternatives – seems a likely place to start in developing that recognition.

The chapter utilizes disparate examples that have a dual purpose. First, I wish to call into question the primacy of individual over group rights in defining what is an issue for ethics and second, I wish to show that the consequences of failing to create an ethics which expands to include groups may be profoundly unhealthy for us all. The examples I have drawn upon are intentionally disparate and may seem to be unconnected to one another – at least initially. This is simply because the domains from which the examples are drawn are not conventionally connected within the culture from which Western ethics and medicine derive. However, following the critical view of culture as obscuring certain connections from view, this way of handling the issue of a constrained ethics seems to me to be a highly appropriate manner in which to expand our conceptual view.

The chapter begins with two examples – the death of one little Mexican girl living in the United States, and a statistical profile of the deaths of a great many Native Canadian children. These deaths are drawn from the lives of impoverished individuals living within groups where the dominant culture of those observing and depicting their plight obscures the issues of social justice and inequity via their representation of culture. In both of these examples culture is trivialized in some manner. Between examples 1 and 2 – the individual and the statistical – I have inserted a brief summary of the major preoccupations of ethics within biomedicine over the last several decades. The placement of this summary between the example of an individual death and the collective deaths of many children means it is meant to be read parenthetically. The main concerns of such a delimited ethics do not touch upon the collective lives of such impoverished children, so it can not adequately frame the individual death of a child living in poverty as due to anything except the culture of the child herself. The second set of examples (3 and 4) deal with the moral implications of the limits imposed by the blinders of a science which does not see itself as culturally situated. These implications are illustrated by the failure of the "objective" concept of post-traumatic stress disorder to differentiate between victims and perpetrators and by the role that the cultural construction of menopause by biomedicine plays in the subordination of women. In these examples the culture of the "expert" obscures certain relations of power from view. Example 5 deals with the role that some core cultural notions underlying

Western biomedical and economic models have played in the rapid evolution of antibiotic resistant bacteria. The last example (6) deals with the deeply problematic view of death in the West that underscores activities which, although they may extend individual lives, ironically may hasten our collective demise. This is discussed as part of our metaphorical "war on disease" which pits humanity against nature, and hence ultimately against itself. In my view, the ethical implications of this are profound.

Culture can be thought of as a broad and deep influence on all human behaviour that is simultaneously personal and social with implications for our species as a whole. The greatest impact of the concept of culture therefore comes not from its application to others in narrow and controlled cross-cultural comparisons of certain domains, but from a clear recognition that it applies profoundly to the lives of those doing work in all aspects of scholarship itself. Culture can not be reduced to a manipulated variable called "cultural beliefs" without considerable collateral damage being done to the people to whom the narrowed concept is applied. In a narrow construction of culture as a residual and manipulated category, the subject population (patients or clients) have "health care beliefs" (culture), while professionals are the bearers of Medicine – a supposedly value-free entity which is valourized as entirely "good" and objectively "true" (science). In the many cross-cultural health care contexts of international development, immigrant and refugee issues, or the struggles of indigenous people around the world, this rapidly becomes a case of "Western minds and foreign bodies" (Hepburn 1992, 59). This is where healthy rationalism is expected to triumph over ignorance and disease because biomedicine is believed to be neutral, scientific, and an objective description of reality uninfluenced by social processes. What should concern us deeply is that this widespread view is not recognized as part of the reproduction of inequity ... including inequities in the provision of health care itself. We also need to question how a too narrowly focused medical ethics might contribute to this process. Let me give you an example of othering – a unilateral ascription of a subjective culture to others which implies a more neutral understanding on the part of an observer with pretensions to objectivity (in this case, a journalist).

Example 1: The death of Sandra Navarrete

(from Chavez, Flores, and Lopez-Garza 1992, 6-7)

> On March 28, 1989, five-year-old Sandra Navarrete died of chicken pox, a childhood disease that is rarely fatal in the United States. Her parents, recent undocumented immigrants from Mexico, did not seek medical care for Sandra until it was too late for successful intervention. Their comments indicated that they did not seek care because they did not know where to go,

they did not speak English, and they had little money (Jones and Reyes 1989:II,1). A few days after this occurred, I received a phone call from a reporter who asked me, "What is it about Mexican culture that prevented Sandra's parents from taking her to get health care?"

Like the reporter who telephoned Leo Chavez in this example, researchers from biomedicine interested in cultural pluralism and health issues often operationalize and greatly restrict the notion of culture by defining it as "a collection of 'cultural beliefs' assessed through questionnaires containing one or two items concerning respondents' ideas about health" (Millard 1992, 4). The resultant trivialization of culture as unarticulated elements of traditions to which others blindly adhere nicely deflects our attention from our own assumptions about knowledge and how these "lie at the heart of contested domains concerning responsibilities, rights, authority, and power" (Millard 1992, 4). Clearly, Sandra Navarrete did not die of either chicken pox or her parents' health care beliefs; she died because her family is desperately poor and isolated. They are impoverished because they are part of a large group of undocumented and unorganized Mexican labourers exploited to keep the California agricultural and textile industries profitable. A broader understanding of culture would allow us to be interested primarily with the web of economic and political relations that subordinate the Navarrete family, with their despair, and the experience of serious illness that emanates from these. It should also bring into sharp relief a question which I would take as central to our concerns – whether the lack of access to care experienced by the Navarrete family is not also a matter which biomedical ethics should more forcefully address. Because Sandra Navarrete and her family are members of a group called "illegals" in the United States, they are defined as a social problem and their lack of access to care understood to be largely unavoidable. Recently this perspective may have expanded to view the provision of care as unwarranted as well. For example, the state of California recently moved to legislate against the rights of such "illegal" children even to attend schools.

Individual-oriented hospital-based ethics has little to say about the Navarrete family, but perhaps it should. What inhibits this discussion? What role does the restriction of notions of culture to a few questions in a medical history or to several variables on a needs assessment questionnaire play in the death of Sandra Navarrete and the suffering of people like her? To begin addressing these questions, we may briefly summarize the thrust of most bioethical concerns over the past several decades. I wish to emphasize that we should understand these as broadly defined concerns of our dominant cultural elite, that is, as ideological productions rather than the uncontested and distilled truths of logic and science.

If Sandra Navarrete's death is not construed as an ethical issue, what is?

Fox (1990, 202) outlines three distinct phases in the evolution of bioethics in the United States, to which we in Canada are also heir. I have appended some significant social and demographic commentaries to his categories.

Bioethics preoccupations of the last few decades

Late-1960s to mid-1970s: Preoccupation with informed consent from human subjects involved in scientific research

These continue to be important issues but they have shifted away from concern with individuals who may be easily exploited (prisoners, children, incompetent aged, mentally and physically handicapped) to the ramification of experiments with genes and frozen embryos, and fetal tissues (culminating in a National Commission for the Protection of Human Subjects of Biomedical and Behavioral Research, est. 1978). This period was consistent with wider societal shifts from concern with deviance to a legal approach to individual rights which preoccupied North Americans at the time. The rights of those living in institutions was of primary concern, the civil rights of those living outside institutions was restricted largely to acts of job discrimination, and did not extend to economic exploitation.

Mid-1970s to mid-1980s: Concern expanded to involve definitions of life, death, and personhood

It should also be noted that the demographic underpinning of these concerns reflects a middle-aged "baby boom" generation simultaneously coming to terms with children and aging/dying parents. The issues of life, death, and personhood reflect everything from the meaning of senile dementia to abortion but are also consistent with the growing commodification of people and their parts. (The President's Commission for the Study of Ethical Problems in Medicine and Biomedical and Behavioural Research was established in 1981.)

Mid-1980s to present: Discussion of cost containment in health care and the allocation of scarce medical resources

This is consistent with wider concerns about high taxes and deficit financing of government debt in an aging population during a period of perceived economic recession. Obviously, these have gained attention and are part of the same bioethical discourse to which we contribute here, and they are part of a broader discussion that includes the death of Sandra Navarrete.

All of the above concerns mirror both technological shifts in biomedicine and alterations in the economic circumstances of an aging population. Marshall (1992) summarizes this nicely as a major interest throughout recent years concerning the nature of personhood. When does individual life begin and end? To a great extent bioethical concern embodies a fundamental concern of our culture, which is to gain personal control over "events that accentuate individual powerlessness" (Marshall 1992, 51). This is true of everything from weight control and associated disorders (e.g. anorexia nervosa) through cosmetic surgery, to the aging process, and especially to death itself. Individual powerlessness is a bleak feature of life in an industrial society that is, ironically, maintained by emphasizing the rights of individuals without acknowledging the importance of group processes in supporting and maintaining those rights. Weakening or even severing the social bonds that might truly grant individuals some measure of power and efficacy in their lives does this. There is also a fundamental contradiction here that stems from advances in medical control, which leads to great ambivalence on the part of the general public. Biotechnology may grant medical science increasingly finer control over the time of death, or the beginning of life, but it simultaneously denies it to patients and their families.

The prevailing ethos of North American jurisprudence, bioethics, marketing, business, and entertainment are all highly similar. As Fox suggests, "the conceptual framework of bioethics has accorded paramount status to the value complex of individualism, underscoring the principles of individual rights, autonomy, self-determination, and their legal expression in the jurisprudential notion of privacy" (1990, 206). There are probably never clear answers to problematic situations involving great pain and suffering, medical uncertainty, and cultural complexity; where individuals are at odds and their rights and obligations collide. However,

> In these situations, rationalistic thinking and a deductive, utilitarian orientation to problem solving provide an illusion of objectivity and logic. Informed by the legacy of Cartesian duality, the analytic style of bioethics contributes to a distancing of moral discourse from the complicated human settings and interactions within which moral dilemmas are culturally constructed, negotiated and lived. In this discourse, issues of personhood, body parts, organ replacements, genetic cloning, and the like are confronted as abstractions rather than experienced realities. (Marshall 1992, 52)

The dilemmas most often defined as moral ones in this discourse are restricted to issues of individual control and rights, while social justice generally gets short shrift. What happens to collectivities in this discourse, particularly where many children like Sandra Navarrete living in marginalized groups die of similarly preventable diseases that are a product of exploitation and poverty?

Example 2: The configuration of mortality and ethics:
Native health in Canada

Concerns over when life begins and ends, the moral quandaries associated with placing baboon organs into human beings, and the future sex lives of frozen fetuses have preoccupied parts of both our scientific and ethical communities. However, they have not proved to be of all-consuming interest in the rest of the world. In Islamic countries, for example, these are widely viewed as the decadent and absurd cultural obsessions of the self-absorbed infidel West. To critics within, these cultural preoccupations are akin to the number of angels that can dance on the head of a pin. What certain cultural obsessions (the sex of our unborn children, the exact moment of our departure from life) reveal is a profound concern with the individual divorced from the social domain where meaning is created. After all, we are dealing with what is personhood on the margins of social life: those pre-persons nearing birth and those becoming post-persons during the process of dying. I think that these preoccupations are configured by the concerns of a mainly urban, predominantly white, and economically privileged segment of the population. There is a powerful demographic and political dynamic underlying all these concerns.

For example, when one compares the population structure of Natives in British Columbia, Canada (non-status Indians) with that of the rest of the province, one notes that the Native population is far younger and has almost no population of seniors when compared with the rest of British Columbians. The non-Native population contains a very large segment of the population in the over 65 years cohort. This latter population is almost completely urban, is mainly white, intensively utilizes hospitals, and is generally far wealthier than their Native counterparts. Much of the actual practice of medical ethics concerns the latter stages of life and is taken up with this wealthier urban white population, and large expenditures of public funds are associated with them. Yet, the mortality statistics for Aboriginal people indicate that a much poorer health status rooted in limited access exists for them. I suggest this is further constrained by a set of beliefs and practices which define their suffering, like Sandra Navarrete's, as a social problem surrounded by an aura of inevitability.[2]

The fact that the Native population is much younger stems from the appalling mortality experienced by the group from birth onwards. The relatively younger Aboriginal population is far more than a reflection of higher birth rates; it exists because the rest of the potential age pyramid has been eroded by constantly higher mortality from just about every cause we have managed to study. Indeed, when one measures this in terms of a comparative statistic known as "potential years life lost standardized rates", one finds that the Native population of British Columbia (whether male or female) loses more than three times as many years as the rest of the population from all sources combined. Particularly startling are the measured rates of Sudden Infant Death Syndrome (SIDS).

There are many risk factors associated with deaths of all infants in their first year, clustering around the fourth and fifth month of life (smoking, low birth weight, maternal anaemia, youth of mother, alcohol and drug use, single status, and lower socio-economic status). The last of these, poverty, is implicated in virtually all of the others, because poverty too often means inadequate maternal nutrition, absent partners, despair, and sometimes addiction. If this childhood and maternal poverty is where the higher mortality trajectory begins in Native populations, then we must wonder why this is not of greater concern to the world of biomedical ethics.

Of course, the Native population is far more rural and has poorer access to care, maternity programs, and all manner of public support. But more particularly, relatively little money is actually expended upon them compared to the dominant groups in Canadian society. To reduce mortality in the first year of life means focusing on social supports for mothers, increased educational opportunities, as well as jobs and income for partners. These are all public health issues; they are deeply social and embedded within a fabric of systemic racism and economic neglect. To deal with these problems in ethical terms means conceptualizing and using an expanded notion of group rights. To understand why they are not now broadly configured as ethical issues we must also look deeply into the culture of the dominant group in Canadian society. We do not need yet another superficial set of generalizations about the culture of Native people that becomes just another way to blame the victims for their problems. We certainly need to understand why this sadly graphic illustration of disastrous and appallingly high numbers of dead Native babies is not in the spotlight for medical ethics. I suggest it will have to become so if we are ever to develop cross-cultural ethics in medicine and health care that deal with more than the pre-occupations of the most powerful cultural groups in our plural society.

The Canadian example of high mortality among Native peoples repeats itself around the globe with colonized populations of indigenous people everywhere. Typically, the leading causes of death in such populations are: 1) circulatory diseases, particularly non-insulin dependent diabetes (NIDDM), associated with loss of land and resources, relocation, and dietary shifts from varied high protein/low carbohydrate diets to limited low protein/high carbohydrate diets (Hefernen 1996; Hopkinson, Stephenson and Turner 1996); 2) violence (including suicide) and accidents, often associated with poverty, substance abuse, and a history of residential school systems and missionization (Cooper 1996, Wade 1996); 3) high rates of untreated infections associated with poor housing, poor diet, lack of access to care, and isolation. Elliott and Foster (1996) depict this situation for Australia, Canada, and New Zealand using data compiled by Shah and Johnson (1992). They show that death from neoplasms (cancers) are roughly the same for each group and much lower than the leading causes of death for each respective group. Cancer kills mainly in older age categories and relatively few of these people ever reach anything like old age (Hislop and Band 1996).

What kind of distractions and enthusiasms contribute to the political economy and limited attention span of a world filled with starving children living in abject poverty who die in droves of common childhood diseases like chicken pox; their suffering somehow construed as inevitable? Their deaths have somehow become too easily viewed as the sadly unavoidable product of cultural inadequacy and degradation brought on by a mixture of corruption, warlords, and poor hygiene. They are not often viewed as a creation of international agribusiness and forestry operations which have alienated much of the world's food producing/yielding lands in less than a century and turned them into coffee, chocolate, citrus, tea, poppy, coca, copra, sisal, cotton, timber, or other plantations. Neither is the destruction of food species habitats by rapacious mining and manufacturing industries generally seen as causal. My point is simply that it is rather easy to do this if we insist that our most powerful science (medicine) and our reified market (economics) are both value free and objective. Other people's cultural realities are reduced to a few beliefs which must be surmounted in order to provide them with hegemonic ideas of "modern" health care while simultaneously moving them away from kinship-based collective respon-sibilities and into the free market system as entrepreneurial individuals. That these are both assimilationist and neocolonial ideas is simply too obvious to need much elaboration, but that they are deeply connected to one another is rarely mentioned (Bodley 1985, 1988, 1990). Certainly they represent a basic issue for cross-cultural ethics.

Example 3: The problematic concept of "post-traumatic stress disorder"

It is generally assumed in psychiatry that Western diagnostic categories and standards of measurement are scientific and hence minimally affected by cultural values. That this is simply a category fallacy can be well understood through a critical examination of so-called post-traumatic stress disorder, or PTSD as it is most commonly known. The symptoms of this "disorder" are well known and need no elaboration here, but one wonders how we can claim that the same terminology applies equally to the victims of torture and the torturers themselves? How is it that Vietnam War veterans and Vietnamese refugees both have PTSD? Those who survived a catastrophic earthquake and those who lived through the process of "ethnic cleansing" in Bosnia are said to suffer in the same way in a common syndrome (Young 1988, 1992, Madaakasira and O'Brien 1987). When we focus on healing, which is an interpersonal process, it becomes clear that whether people suffer as a result of human brutality or from natural disasters must play a role in the therapeutic process. It is, after all, the bonds of human trust that must be refashioned in the former case. Including the tortured with their tormentors under the same rubric begs all kinds of questions about what is obfuscated through a medicalized acronym like "PTSD". In this instance, as in the earlier discussion of agribusiness, the culture of the observer tends to obscure something important from our view – human agency in the creation of immense suffering. To be sure, soldiers are brutalized by war, but categorizing them after the fact together with the civilians of a country to which they were sent as an invasion force removes the war itself from moral view. It also excludes those who send the youth of a country into war from critical view altogether. Who killed all those Americans listed on the War Memorial in Washington, those who shot them, or those who sent them there? Even the term "natural disaster" is problematic; it draws attention away from the poor housing in which people are forced to live and relegates the high toll from earthquakes to the realm of the inevitable, rather than situating it in the universe of the preventable.

This leads us into an analytic view of culture which emphasizes what is hidden by culture as well as what is revealed by it. Now,

> the emphasis has shifted from what culture allows and enables people to see, feel and do, to what it restricts and inhibits them from seeing, feeling and doing. Further, although it is agreed that culture powerfully constitutes the reality that actors live in, this reality is looked upon with critical eyes: why this one and not some other? And what sorts of alternatives are people being disabled from seeing? (Ortner 1984, 152)

This is not simply the conventional Marxist formula of mystified power relations; Ortner implies something much more personal and perceptual. If we have forgone collective responsibility in the world in favour of individual protection from liability, then is this because we fail to recognize our own beliefs as cultural productions while insisting that others' problems stem solely from forces at work in *their* cultures?

The "aura of factuality" (after Geertz, 1973) in culture which is conveyed by medical research and practice must become the object of scrutiny precisely because it so powerfully asserts itself as having reached some sort of unassailable scientific bedrock truth. Critical analysis begins with the observation that, as Keesing (1987, 161) put it, "Cultures are webs of mystification as well as signification". This mystification only begins to dissolve when we come to understand that, as Alan Young succinctly puts it, "in industrial societies the most powerful ideological practices are ones which claim that their facts are non-ideological because they are scientific" (1983, 209).

Example 4: Aging and the fallacy of reproductive "loss" in menopause

It takes what Martin (1987, 52) describes as a "jolt" to better understand the "contingent nature" of biomedical description and analysis, and this can happen when one's own assumptions are revealed in another cultural context. For many anthropologists, working in cultures other than their own with older individuals as cultural interpreters has revealed, quite unbidden, the nature of age stratification in their own societies. This stratification and stigmatization of the elderly is grounded in an ideology of aging within biomedicine itself as the medicalization of old age. The process is particularly gendered and simultaneously yields the view that men inevitably die young due to constitutional deficiencies and that women live longer but essentially unproductive lives. Both of these are ideological constructions based upon social forces at work upon men and women in industrial societies. The discussion here relates to women's health but a similar deconstruction of men's socialization into high stress and dangerous careers and early mortality experiences propped up by an ideology which normalizes this as essentially male is easily conceived.

Martin (1987) deconstructs the representations of women's bodies found in medical textbooks and concludes that several powerful metaphors of women's bodies permeate these textbooks and that they are cloaked in scientific (supposedly value-free or neutral) terminology. Martin finds one metaphor employed throughout these texts is that the female body is geared to "production" (not really reproduction, I would add) and consists of a control hierarchy which begins to falter and break down. The image is identical with that of our economic system. In menopause, she writes, "what is being described is a break-down of a system of authority ... at every point in this system, functions "fail" and "falter". Follicles, for example, "fail to muster strength to reach ovulation. As functions fail, so do the members of the system decline" (1987, 42). The key to the metaphor, as Martin sees it, is "functionlessness". She concludes, "these images frighten us in part because in our stage of advanced capitalism, they are close to a reality we find difficult to see clearly: broken down hierarchy and organizational members who no longer play their designated parts". I would add that outside the body the hierarchy which is breaking down is also one of male authority, and the members no longer playing their designated parts are (mainly) women. Not only, as Martin forcefully concludes, is the body described in a way that props up a view of women as defined solely by their reproductive function, but this is done in a manner which strongly implies that menopause is a negative experience and that post-menopausal women do not have an economic role to play – being broken parts, as it were, and viewed as emotionally unstable ones at that. Such a negative evaluation of identity and slim prospects for the future can easily lead to anger, which is transformed into a symptom and called pre-menstrual syndrome (PMS).

A considerable literature exists on post-menopausal women's lives outside of the mainstream of industrial capitalism. In Oceanic societies, after women stop having children, they enter the domain of political leadership. A considerable number of Oceanic peoples have older women and younger men – often their sons – serve as political leaders. Many old men retire to a life socializing with one another, caring for grandchildren, and fishing. The change of role from that of a person prohibited via various taboos (centred on menstruation and fertility) from playing political roles is essentially validated for women by menopause and the clarity of mind it is said to bring (Brown and Kern 1985). This reinterpretation of what menstrual taboos mean has also been extended to various Native American groups (Underhill 1965; Powers 1980; Wright 1982; Buckley 1982). What then, happens to the so-called symptoms of menopause and PMS in such societies?

There is a considerable literature that has shown that the experience of menopause is quite variable and, not surprisingly, related to the position of women in particular societies (Lock 1993; Davis 1996). Menopause and PMS are relatively culture-bound expressions of so-called symptoms operating in societies where change in fertility has long been construed as a loss of fertility, i.e. as a deficit. Most disturbingly, even though there is little evidence for menopause and PMS as universal experiences of women, negative connotations and readings of the change of life can be introduced by what is essentially medical propaganda and a changing view of women associated with the spread of biomedicine (Davis, 1996, 75).[3]

There is another approach to this issue that complements both the analysis of language afforded by deconstruction and the cross-cultural research into roles and symptoms. This challenge to medical orthodoxy is particularly ironic because it challenges biomedicine on something like its own territory as essentially an uncritical and culture-bound form of folk biology of the West. What is the biological relationship between fertility, physical decline, and death?

Evolutionary anthropologists, zoologists, and primatologists have long noted that fertility is not directly or invariably related to systemic decline and mortality in animals. At one end of a spectrum, some animals essentially spawn and die in such a manner that the two processes are entwined. The entire digestive tract of some migratory fish (salmon for example) is reabsorbed and energy and space directed into reproduction. At the other end of the spectrum, highly social animals can have a prolonged post-fertile stage in their lives. Interestingly, in human beings and other highly social primates, this stage may even exceed in duration the period of socialization of the young of the species.

There also exists an abundance of information on child care and provisioning in many groups of food foragers which shows that after infants begin to walk with confidence, they often become the charges of the oldest generation. The parental generation is often busy acquiring food – indeed, they may be the only ones allowed to hunt and gather because the activity is considered to be polluting in some fashion. Turnbull's (1983) description of Mbuti society vividly illustrates this and adds yet another ironic element; it is the youth and the elderly among the Mbuti who are allowed to make political commentary and reprimand the middle-aged adults for their anti-social behaviour.

Did natural selection play a role in creating both a long period of socialization and a long post-fertility stage in the lives of women? Are the two not rather directly related each producing the other? Viewed in this way, the negative construction of post-menopausal life becomes, instead, a species-specific adaptive attribute of human beings. To construe menopause as a "loss" obscures what might be understood far more profoundly as the way our species gained its most defining attribute: culture. The evolutionary development of culture depended on an adaptation that allows for considerable post-reproductive life, particularly among women. Such a view of post-fertile life span suggests that it is a highly evolved characteristic and part of what has made us into homo sapiens: cultural knowledge shared among three generations rather than simple survival techniques transmitted between two. What kind of an ideology operates in such a way that something as profoundly human as the collective evolutionary gain of culture as a species attribute can be viewed as inevitable individual loss? It must be a powerful ideology asserting a form of truth that it is incontestable and exclusively individuated.

The evolutionary perspective just introduced allows us to examine another critically important area where the weight of the scales of eternal justice have tipped so far towards individual rights over group rights that I fear we may have endangered ourselves as a species.

Example 5: Pharmaceuticals and the ultimate iatrogenesis

(From Stephenson, 1986, 48-50; 1989; 1991.)

As almost every student of pathogenesis and infectious disease has come to understand, over time natural selection tends to favour the less virulent forms of any particular pathogenic organism. This is simply because the most virulent forms wipe themselves out when they kill their hosts. For example, we can see that many pathogenic relationships between organisms which afflict mammals are now carried rather benignly by reptiles and birds who have had much longer periods of evolutionary time to come to terms with them. The greatest scourge of humankind since the advent of agriculture in central Africa, plasmodium (malaria), is an example of this.

> A corollary of our discussion thus far is that a well-adapted "healthy" parasite is one which has increased its potential for survival by not killing the host. In evolutionary terms, this means that older parasites are often highly complex in their interaction with their hosts, and while they may kill some, particularly children and older people, they debilitate many. They also will have evoked an adaptive response on the part of humans which is genetic in those areas where the disease is endemic. (Stephenson 1986, 49-50)

What do we accomplish when we indiscriminately apply broad-spectrum antibiotics to mild infections in otherwise healthy individuals? We now recognize that this creates a hot-house environment for the breeding of increasingly virulent forms of the infectious diseases originally targeted. Moreover, we also disrupt many other unintended targets with pharmaceuticals, causing them to evolve in completely unpredictable and even potentially lethal ways. This process of pharmaceutical driven micro-evolution of virtually all bacteria and some viruses is one we blithely call "medicine". One is given to wonder at the ultimate wisdom of this and to ponder the role that individual rights ascendant over collective responsibilities may play in ever trying to remove so-called "modern medicine" from this nasty evolutionary *cul de sac.*

Disturbingly virulent forms of old diseases (and perhaps a few entirely new diseases) are increasingly the legacy of the era of the "magic bullet" (Stephenson 1989; 1991). But most insidiously, the pharmaceutical industry is unlikely to change this situation for the simple reason that a positive feed-back loop links their profit motives to epidemiological imperatives when so-called "new" diseases arise or resistant bacteria evolve. Quite simply, a larger potential market arrives with every resistant strain that appears. Our pharmaceutical industry then appears to contain a fundamental iatrogenic contradiction, which is obscured by common parlance surrounding the terms "medicine" and "cure". After all, we say that "medicines cure disease", we do not conventionally say they "cause" it! A more culturally situated

evolutionary and economic understanding of the Western antibiotic pharmacopoeia rooted in social costs as opposed to individual gains suggests
something very different. Each new generation of antibiotics increases
pathogenic resistance in a downward spiral spreading death and destruction
in its wake along with a generous bonus of increasing dividends for wealthy
individuals and corporations.

> What does this dismal scenario entail for either the concept of culture, or
> medical ethics? I think it means leaving behind the deeply mistaken
> Cartesian notion that biology and culture are not intrinsically linked in
> human experience. Humans have blundered into the biological realm while
> under the illusion that they were "controlling disease" through the sheer
> brilliance of their culturally-based superiority.

In his influential work, *The Predicament of Culture*, Clifford (1988)
concludes that the idea of coherent "cultures" is deeply problematic.
According to Clifford, anthropologists (among others) have generally used
the culture concept to imagine a world of neatly bounded, internally
"coherent", aesthetically "balanced" collective entities. However, such a
concept,

> contain[s] and domesticate[s] heteroglossia. In a world with too many voices
> speaking all at once, a world where syncretism and parodic invention are
> becoming the rule ... it becomes increasingly difficult to attach human
> identity and meaning to a coherent "culture" or "language" (Clifford 1988,
> 95).

Thus Clifford rejects essentialist models of culture and identity. Culture is
not located within a group, just as identity does not inhere in individual
human beings. Rather, culture and identity happen between people: "we
should attempt to think of cultures not as organically united or traditionally
continuous but ... as negotiated, present processes" (Clifford 1988, 273). He
concludes that the "deeply compromised idea" of culture must be "replaced
by some set of relations that preserves the concept's differential and
relativist functions and that avoids the positing of cosmopolitan essences and
human common denominators" (1988, 274-75).

This newer formulation of culture must itself be multivocal and grounded
in experience as opposed to defined in universalist terms. Such a
conceptualization may allow for intercultural understanding as opposed to
cross-cultural studies. Yet we must also caution that Clifford's argument
about culture as a loose construct containing internal contradictions and
incoherence is mainly an analytical perspective informed by the chaotic
aspects of social life. From a more localized and grounded ethnographic
point of view many newly consolidated identities – sexual, ethnic, and
cultural – are also continuously being asserted and the symbols used to unite

these identities in the political domain are created against a backdrop of alienation and a human need for meaning and consistency. Thus, there are forces pushing the other way too – towards homogeneity and consolidation in a specified place and time. One has only to think of many ethnic nationalistic movements around the world to see that the creation of culture is a process of fusion as well as fission.

If the most salient lesson to be drawn from Clifford's critique is that culture is a process occurring between people(s), then the transmission and creation of both illnesses and health care are also cultural processes occurring between us. How can this plural perspective inform our view of the meaningfulness of mortality, and hence lend meaning to life?

Case 6: Mortality and death: the dance of measurement and meaning

Consider for a moment the recent rather surreal court cases of a physician in the United States who has been given the moniker "Dr Death" by the public and the tabloid media. Dr Kavorkian has invented a machine that allows his clientele – mainly individuals with mortal illnesses – to push a button, leading to the release of a lethal substance through an I.V. As a person who has witnessed the deaths and attended funerals of a number of people in various cultural contexts (Hutterian, Cree, Haida, and Dutch), this has always struck me as a particularly absurd medical appropriation of a natural process. What is it about industrial medicine that has made people feel that they require this kind of assistance? In many cultures, people can often die more or less when they want to because they stop eating and taking fluids and their desire to do so is respected. If one takes in no water for a couple of days, one dies. Not only do people in many cultural groups know when and how to die, but cats and dogs often manage this too – if we let them.

The variation in mortality experiences of Hutterites as these relate to aging, sex roles, and fertility (Stephenson 1991; 1985; 1983) are particularly relevant here. The Hutterites are a communal farming people who share many religious and cultural similarities to the Amish and Mennonites. They dwell mainly in the Canadian prairie provinces and several northern plains states of the U.S., but do not share a similar life expectancy pattern to that of the rest of North America. They may be the only known group in the industrialized world where men and women die at about the same age – indeed men may even outlive women by an average of about six months. In trying to understand how this comes about I have had most of my notions about death itself challenged. I have concluded (in contrast to the proponents of the doctrine of specific aetiology) that people almost never die of any one underlying cause but of multiple factors. Whenever a specific cause of death has been sought for in epidemiological studies of Hutterite women, it has only been found that they have fewer deaths from that cause than would be expected. The Hutterites die earlier from less of just about everything than does much of Canadian society in the prairie region where they dwell. They have lower rates of cancer, in particular. What do they die from?

Early researchers concluded that the high numbers of births per woman (a measure called parity) was responsible through some sort of systemic weakening of their bodies. This hypothesis went untested for about thirty years and derives from the same perspective which Martin so successfully deconstructed. I should also point out that large families are often considered to be irresponsible and unhealthy by the social class and society from which the researchers themselves were drawn. Parkinson (1981) finally showed that there are no statistical or clinical data to support the parity hypothesis. Indeed, Hutterian women with the largest number of children appear to live slightly longer on average, although the age difference is not particularly significant. Long-term ethnographic fieldwork suggested instead that many Hutterian women probably die earlier than non-Hutterite counterparts of multiple sub-clinical cardiovascular conditions within a context where death is not feared and where dying becomes a long drawn out social process that involves being visited by dispersed daughters. In short, death does not mean the same thing to Hutterites as it has meant to medical researchers.

For the Hutterites dying is a normal, inevitable process which makes one the focus of community attention and love. It concludes a period of relative isolation from one's dead kin and friends and transports one to the realm of eternal perfect communal living (heaven) while ending a life of increasing travail and isolation. To many researchers, however, death is generally the enemy; it is, if not entirely preventable, then something to be indefinitely postponed. Any conventional demographic or epidemiological use of mortality statistics to try to either evaluate or prolong life in the Hutterite colonies is likely doomed to failure. Hutterites tend to greet death with hope rather than fear and prefer a prolonged deathbed to a sudden departure. Just how does one do comparative epidemiology when the major variables for severity of expression of symptoms and even mortality itself are embedded in cultural values that evaluate pain and death very differently from the way the researcher does? Have we made of death such a fearsome "enemy" that we no longer know it as a universal and normal experience? In ethical terms, how would we approach doing health promotion with people like the Hutterites? These are people for whom a better quality of life may be desirable, but desire for a longer life is not necessarily a valid proposition and for whom death is normal and has not been medicalized.

Conclusion: the *"war on disease"*: who are the victims?

Recently I have come to view much of industrial medicine as founded to a great extent on culture specific metaphorical notions of a moral war. The working conditions of almost any emergency ward in a major city in the industrialized world tend strongly to reinforce such a view. People maimed in accidents or assaulted by those around them swamp emergency wards. The case load of traumatic injury is so heavy in many of these institutions that the same kinds of medicine (triage, gallows humour, etc.) as prevails in war are found in them. The many television programs based on the lives and work of people in the E.R. at hospitals both reflect and to a certain extent validate this perception. Many physicians undertake their basic training in such circumstances, but neither they or other health professionals receive much training in public health and they know little of the culturally diverse populations they must serve. When this (understandable) siege mentality is extended into the realm of chronic problems, however, disease becomes the enemy instead of the poverty, ignorance, and neglect which produce it.

Although our many disease conditions are "targeted" by drugs, "bombarded" with X-rays, and "operations" performed to remove various "invasions" of our personal landscapes, our experience of this war is deeply problematic. The perceived enemy is, as always, small and utilizes guerrilla tactics to which we, in the ranks of industrial medicine, are extremely vulnerable.

In this metaphorical war against disease, the historical significance of our allies – medical technology and "civilized" culture – has been greatly overestimated. Perhaps our view of disease grows out of the assertion of almost complete power over the lives of others established during wars of colonial expansion. This was really a conquest by disease more than any form of military or cultural superiority. As McNeil (1976; 1979) has shown, the disease load harboured by civilization has been its major weapon during colonial expansion. Epidemics of diseases causing herd immunity in adult survivors are maintained in large, dense populations via the annual infection of large numbers of children. These "childhood" infectious diseases evolved from herd and flock animals along with agriculture and animal husbandry. They were (and are) devastating to smaller societies when both children and adults become simultaneously infected. Not only are adults far more seriously symptomatic, but they cannot care for their infected children which leads to exceedingly high overall mortality.

The political advantage won for Western medicine in the colonial encounter between resistant adult Europeans and diseased and dying indigenous peoples around the world is difficult to overestimate. Both parties appear to have attributed notions of superiority (cultural and racial) to immune Europeans. Paradoxically, the greatest initial advantage Europeans had over smaller cultures and their medical practices was not their medicines, it was their diseases (Cohen 1989). Many still live with the illusion, however, that it was a superior culture in the form of technology and medicine that gained for the West much of the world. The illusion that the West is all powerful and that the residual dangers to our health come from the colonized (rather than the other way around) still holds sway in popular opinion.

To summarize, much of Western medical ethics has been framed by a set of cultural themes from which I suggest we must begin to break away in the interest of global health and the cross-cultural experience which increasingly forms our lives.

1) Individual demands have generally been valued at the expense of group rights. Put in another way, our notion seems to be that individuals have rights; groups have responsibilities to individuals, and it is almost never the other way around. Since culture is quintessentially a group concept with ramifications for individuals, then a cross-cultural medical ethics will of necessity have to move beyond the dimension of individual entitlements and rights and towards some way of addressing the rights of groups.

2) In many developed countries, a large population cohort of elderly individuals obsessed with youth and phobic about death utilizes vast amounts of health care resources in the last months of life. Medicalization can make old age a nightmare for many seniors and their families while simultaneously diverting limited resources from prevention of problems among marginalized minorities. A generalized extreme fear of death (thanataphobia) also wreaks havoc with the normal aging process for both women and men and even distorts our understanding of what makes us human...the long post-fertile life stage which allowed culture to evolve in the first place. A critical approach to this means shifting the concerns of medical ethics from the tangle of individual rights at life-end stages dominated by technology towards group processes that promote prevention and acceptance of life and death as normal events.

3) Competition is pervasive and actually believed to be the universal fountainhead of individual creativity in a globalizing economy. This particular ideological permutation of capitalism creates adversarial relationships and dilemmas where many solutions must be co-operative. Much discourse in medical ethics takes the narrative form of debate between two sides (a competition) of an issue with a winning position (from which the individual will profit). That this is culturally situated seems obvious; that it often simply reproduces problems rather than finding solutions appears to be almost invisible to the participants.

4) The widespread view of co-operation as a suspect activity that is unnatural, and, at any rate, unattainable in the individual struggle to survive is a corollary of (3). This makes solution oriented programs directed at prevention and promotion in cross-cultural contexts extremely difficult to maintain. Where failure is expected, the economic and structural supports required to achieve success are generally minimized, any consequent failure of co-operative activities is then said to prove the point that was initially presumed. Much inadequate funding for public health initiatives among marginalized groups (the homeless, indigenous groups, etc.) is like this and never moves beyond inadequately funded demonstration projects.

5) The conquest of much of the world by Europeans tends to be viewed as the inevitable result of cultural and technical superiority (including medicine) rather than as the result of diseases transmitted to non-immune populations which killed millions of people between 1500 and 1900. This illusory interpretation of history tends to breed an arrogant and ignorant self-confidence about cultural hegemony and buttresses a supremely over-confident science. Cross-cultural ethics of medicine will have to be vigilant in adopting a more self-critical stance and be able to hear other points of view through a very dense and rather self-congratulatory cultural screen.

All of these points appear to be related to an extraordinary need to exert personal control over events that accentuate individual powerlessness. As such, the actual existence of the collectivities ("we-selves") to which we belong – families, cultures, species – is threatened by an ascendant form of individualism (the "I-self"). This, in my view, leads to neglect of minority groups and to a view of public health that is not constructed or understood in ethical terms. A recent cover of *Life Magazine* asks: "Can We Stop Ageing?". Ironically, one wonders if notions of individual immortality will make us collectively extinct. Our view of our place in the world, of other organisms, like our idea of our place among other peoples, appears to be deeply flawed by the notion that we are incontestably superior beings, with an arsenal at our disposal. Left unchanged, I fear greatly the widespread idea that we must first delay and then choose the time of our going will ultimately hasten our species' departure from the scene. Dreams of immortality are antithetical rather than fundamental to the love and care of others that should be intrinsic to health care and to cross-cultural ethics which could support it. Milan Kundera, in his book *Immortality*, summarizes this nicely:

> The gesture of longing for immortality knows only two points in space: the self here, the horizon far in the distance; only two concepts: the absolute that is the self, and the absolute that is the world. That gesture has nothing in common with love, because the other, the fellow creature, the person between these two poles (the self and the world) is excluded in advance, ruled out of the game, invisible" (Kundera 1990, 211)

Notes

1. I would especially like to thank Caroline Francis of Mahidol University for all her help in the early stages of writing this chapter. Conversations and exchanges of unpublished material about various aspects of these topics with Naomi Adelson, Sharon Koehn, and Margaret Lock have also proved very helpful. All of my colleagues in this enterprise have proven to be interesting and helpful but I am particularly indebted to the graciousness of my Thai hosts while visiting Bangkok in 1995 and to many stimulating conversations with my friend Barry Glickman.

2. See Foster, et al. (1995) for a detailed discussion.

3. Diet is also a largely unexamined factor in the experience of PMS in particular, although its implications for menopause are somewhat better understood. There are many naturally occurring estrogens in plants and there are also numerous human-made products (plastics, herbicides) which mimic estriadol. These forces may influence population specific physiological experiences around reproduction in ways we are only beginning to understand.

References

Bodley, John H. 1985. *Anthropology and Contemporary Human Problems.* 2nd Ed. Mountain View, California: Mayfield.

———. 1988. *Tribal Peoples and Development Issues: A global overview.* Mountain View, California: Mayfield.

———. 1990. *Victims of Progress,* 3rd Ed. Mountain View, California: Mayfield.

Brown, Judith K. and Virginia Kerns, (Eds.). 1985. *In her prime: A new view of middle-aged women.* South Hadley, Mass.: Bergin and Garvey.

Brown, Judith K. 1970 A note on the division of labor by sex. *American Anthropologist* 72 (5):1073-78.

Buckley, Thomas. 1982 Menstruation and the power of Yurok women: Methods in cultural reconstruction. *American Anthropologist* 9 (1):47-61.

Cassirer, E. 1973 *Langue et mythe. À propos des noms de dieux.* Paris: Les Éditions de Minuit.

Chavez, Leo R., T. Flores Estevan, and Marta Lopez-Garza. 1992. Undocumented Latin American immigrants and U.S. health services: An approach to a political economy of utilization. *Medical Anthropology Quarterly* 6, 1:6-26.

Clifford, James. 1988 *The predicament of culture: Twentieth-century ethnography, literature and art.* Cambridge, MA: Harvard University Press.

Cohen, Mark Nathan. 1989. *Health and the rise of civilization.* New Haven: Yale University Press.

Cooper, Mary. 1995 Aboriginal suicide rates: Indicators of needy communities. In *A persistent spirit: Towards understanding Aboriginal health in British Columbia,* ed. Peter H. Stephenson, Susan J. Elliott, Leslie T. Foster, and Jill Harris, 207-222. Victoria: Western Geographical Press.

Davis, Donna. 1996. The cultural constructions of the premenstrual and menopause syndromes. In *Gender and Health: An International Perspective,* ed. Carolyn F. Sargent and Caroline B. Brettell, 57-86. Upper Saddle River, NJ: Prentice Hall.

Foster, L. T., J. Macdonald, T. A.Tuk, S. H. Uh, and D. Talbot. 1995. Native health in British Columbia: A vital statistics perspective. In *A persistent spirit: Towards understanding Aboriginal health in British Columbia*, ed. Peter H. Stephenson, Susan J. Elliott, Leslie T. Foster, and Jill Harris, 43-94. Victoria: Western Geographical Press.

Fox, Renee C. 1990. The evolution of American bioethics: A sociological perspective. In *Social science perspectives on medical ethics*, ed. George Weisz, 201-220. Philadelphia: University of Pennsylvania Press.

Geertz, Clifford. 1973. *The interpretation of cultures*. New York: Basic Books.

Heffernan, M. Clare. 1995. Diabetes and Aboriginal peoples: the Haida Gwaii diabetes project in a global perspective. In *A persistent spirit: Towards understanding Aboriginal health in British Columbia*, ed. Peter H. Stephenson, Susan J. Elliott, Leslie T. Foster, and Jill Harris, 261-296. Victoria: Western Geographical Press.

Hislop, T. G. and Pierre Band. 1995. Epidemiology of cancer in First Nations people in British Columbia. In *A persistent spirit: Towards understanding Aboriginal health in British Columbia*, ed. Peter H. Stephenson, Susan J. Elliott, Leslie T. Foster, and Jill Harris, 249-260. Victoria: Western Geographical Press.

Hepburn, Sharon J. 1988. Western minds, foreign bodies. *Medical Anthropology Quarterly* 2, 1:59-74

Hopkinson, Jennifer, Peter Stephenson, and Nancy J. Turner. 1995 Changing traditional diet and nutrition in Aboriginal peoples of coastal British Columbia. In *A persistent spirit: Towards understanding Aboriginal health in British Columbia*, ed. Peter H. Stephenson, Susan J. Elliott, Leslie T. Foster, and Jill Harris, 129-166. Victoria: Western Geographical Press.

Jones, Lanie, and David Reyes. 1989. Death of 5-year old under investigation. *Los Angeles Times* 4 April:II:1.

Keesing, Roger M. 1974. Theories of culture. *Annual Review of Anthropology* 3: 73-98.

————. 1987. Anthropology as interpretative quest. *Current Anthropology* 28: 161-169.

Kundera, Milan. 1990. *Immortality* New York: Harper.

Lock, Margaret. 1993. *Encounters with ageing: Mythologies of menopause in Japan and North America.* Berkeley: University of California Press.

Madakasira, Sudhakar and Kevin F. O'brien. 1987. Acute posttraumatic stress disorder in victims of natural disaster. *The Journal of Nervous and Mental Disorder* 175: 286-290.

Martin, Emily. 1987. *The woman in the body: A cultural analysis of reproduction*. Boston: Beacon Press.

Marshall, Paricia A. 1992. Anthropology and bioethics. *Medical Anthropology Quarterly* 6, 1:49-73.

McNeil, William. 1976. *Plagues and people*. Garden City, N.Y.: Anchor.

————. 1979. *The human condition*. Princeton, N.J.: Princeton University Press.

Millard, Ann V. 1992. The anthropological analysis of health. *Medical Anthropology Quarterly* 6,1:3-5.

Ortner, Sherry B. 1984. Theory in anthropology since the sixties. *Society for Comparative Study of Society and History* 84: 126-166.

Powers, Marla. 1980. Menstruation and reproduction: An Oglala case. *Signs* 6 (1):54-65

Shah C. P. and R. Johnson. 1992. Comparing health status: Native Peoples of Canada, Aborigines of Australia, and Maoris of New Zealand. *Canadian Family Physician* 38, 1205-1219.

Stephenson, Peter H. 1991. *The Hutterian people: Ritual and rebirth in the evolution of communal life.* Lanham, MD: University Press of America.

————. 1991. Le sida, la syphilis et la stigmatisation: La genèse des politiques et des préjugés. *Anthropologie et Sociétés* 15, 2-3:91-104.

————. 1989. The biological and social dimensions of AIDS: The origin and transmission of a stigmatized virus. *The Advocate: Journal of the Vancouver Bar Association* 47, 1:53-64.

———. 1986. *Medical anthropology*. (Text to accompany 8 one-hour videos). University of Victoria, Victoria, B.C.

———. 1985. Gender, ageing and mortality in Hutterite society: A critique of the doctrine of specific etiology. *Medical Anthropology* 9 (4):355-363.

———. 1983. "He died too quick!": The process of dying in a Hutterian colony. *Omega* 14 (2):127-34

Stephenson, Peter, S. Elliott, L. Foster, and J. Harris (Eds.). 1995. *A persistent spirit: towards understanding Aboriginal health in British Columbia.* Victoria: Western Geographical Press.

Turnbull, Colin. 1983. *The Mubuti Pygmies: change and adaptation.* New York: Holt, Rinehart and Winston.

Underhill, Ruth. 1965 *Red Man's religion*. Chicago: University of Chicago Press.

Wade, Allan. 1996. Resistance knowledges: Therapy with Aboriginal persons who have experienced violence. In *A persistent spirit: Towards understanding Aboriginal health in British Columbia*, ed. Peter H. Stephenson, Susan J. Elliott, Leslie T. Foster, and Jill Harris, 167-106. Victoria: Western Geographical Press.

Wright Anne. 1982. Attitudes towards childbearing and Menstruation among the Navaho. In *Anthropology of human birth*, ed. Margarita Arschwager Kay, 377-394. Philadelphia: F. A. Davis Co.

Young, Alan. 1983. The creation of medical knowledge: Some problems in interpretation. *Social Science and Medicine* 15B: 379-386.

———. 1988. A description of how ideology shapes knowledge of a mental disorder (Post Traumatic Stress Disorder). Paper prepared for conference no. 106, "Analysis in Medical Anthropology", Wenner-Gren For Anthropological Research, Lisbon, Portugal, (March).

———. 1992. Reconstructing rational minds: Psychiatry and morality in the treatment of posttraumatic stress disorder. In *The social construction of illness: Illness and medical knowledge in past and present*, ed. J. Lachumund and G. Stollberg, 115-124. Stuttgart: Franz Steiner Verlag.

Chapter 6
Health, Health Care, and Culture: Diverse Meanings, Shared Agendas

Michael McDonald

Introduction

In this chapter I focus on two important questions that were basic to the investigation of cross-cultural approaches to health care ethics represented in this volume. First of all: What are health, disease, life, and death from the viewpoints of various cultural, religious, and secular perspectives? Secondly: What is it to be a health care provider? – which raises questions about the training and legitimation of providers as well as recipients or patients.

Three basic concepts – *health, health care,* and *culture* – are central to these questions. I will discuss these three concepts in the context of potential and actual conflicts between the multiple perspectives implied in the first question and the kind of shared social agenda implied in development of a cross-cultural approach to health care ethics. On the one hand, if multiple perspectives on health, disease, life, and death are ethically determinative, then it is reasonable to ask how people operating from diverse cultural, religious, and secular perspectives can find a common moral basis for social action, e.g. in the training and legitimation of health care providers or in the development of health care policy in a multicultural state. While prioritizing multiple perspectives lets participating individuals and groups remain true to their own deeply felt values, it seems to leave no principled way of resolving the inevitable differences that will arise in cross-cultural interchanges, particularly in multicultural societies.

On the other hand, if the construction of shared moral agendas around health care prevails, then the multiple cultural, religious, and secular perspectives seem to be subordinated to an arbitrarily selected set of moral values. This achieves social co-ordination at the expense of downgrading deeply felt and even identifying differences (McDonald 1992). It acutely raises the question of whose values are to be regarded as dominant and whose values are to be relegated to subordinate status in drawing up shared social agendas around crucial health care choices.

The central question I will address in this concluding chapter to Part I is: Can health, health care, and culture be construed in ways that allow us to construct an ethics of health care that is sensitive to cultural, religious, and other differences, but still allows for shared normative stances on pressing moral and political choices in and around health care? In other words, is there a way of avoiding an unhappy choice between either respect for cultural differences or the adoption of common moral agendas in health care? The sort of ethics I am seeking in this chapter would be sensitive to the cultural, religious, and other forms of diversity that mark us as socially situated human beings, e.g. as described by Hui in his chapter on Chinese medicine and Ratanakul in his discussion of Buddhism and health. Yet at the same time it would be an ethics that permits us to make progress on cross-cultural issues. It would, for example, help us resist the misuses of cultural labelling that Stephenson describes in the story of Sandra Navarette and to address the issues of racism, sexism, and exploitation that Anderson and Reimer Kirkham explore in their chapter.

Since I use the tools, language, and materials of analytical philosophy to explore the intersection of various conceptualizations of health, health care, and culture, this chapter may strike some readers as rather dry and abstract. Yet I am convinced that the concepts discussed in this chapter are important and need to be understood in order to develop a satisfactory response to the first two research questions. Fortunately, readers of this volume can find a counterbalance to this austere approach to developing a cross-cultural health care ethics in the richly contextualized approaches offered by my colleagues in this volume. Readers should use the chapters such as those offered in Parts II, III, and IV, to test the central ideas I advance in this chapter. Readers should also be cautioned that there are other ways than mine of understanding health, health care, and culture. These are not eternal concepts fixed in a timeless platonic realm of ideas. Rather they must be contextually located.[1]

Health and its negative correlates

My starting point is with a review of recent philosophical debates about the concept of health. In these debates, the main question is meta-ethical: whether health and, by implication, health care are value-free or value-laden concepts.[2] This is a question that has already been given sociological (chapter 4) and anthropological (chapter 5) analysis. In those chapters, the possibility of seeing modern biomedicine as "value free" or "culturally neutral" was thoroughly criticized. Indeed, a unifying thesis of this book is that biomedicine is not objectively neutral but is itself a culture with its own set of values and cultural context. This chapter begins by examining the opposing (and in many quarters the "received") position, namely a "value-free" concept of health and medicine – analysed this time from the perspective of modern Western philosophy.

Is the philosophy of medicine best understood from the perspective of a positivistic (empirical and value-free) philosophy of science or instead from the value-laden perspectives of moral and political philosophy? In more recent years, philosophical discussions about the value-ladenness of health and health care have been joined by political philosophers arguing about the role of the state in providing health care and, particularly in the American context, over whether and to what extent there should state-provided health care, as there is in Canada (see Daniels 1985).

The question of whether health and health care are essentially scientific or ethical constructs has significant practical implications for the delivery of health care in Thailand, Canada, and most modern societies. Many of those involved in providing, consuming, and funding orthodox, biomedically based health care and in the health sciences conceptualize "health" as essentially objective, value free, and best achieved through the efforts of objective and disengaged scientists who find "cures" for various physiological malfunctions (cf. Gordon 1988). That is, they see health care as rooted in the health sciences. On this view, health *care* is seen as the vehicle for delivering health *cures* – cures validated by standard scientific testing (e.g. double blind randomized clinical trials or statistically sound epidemiological studies).

This scientific conceptualization of health is shared by many health practitioners and shapes to a large extent the institutional structures involved in the training, accreditation, and professional organization of health care providers and health scientists nationally and internationally. It also frames the delivery and practice of health care ethics education in Western hospitals, health science faculties, and other health care institutions. More generally, explicit and implicit claims to scientific objectivity form an important aspect of the global process of modernization, in particular, the spread of scientific biomedicine throughout the world. Hence, in trying to develop an adequate cross-cultural approach to health care ethics, it is important to examine the underlying philosophical foundations of these purportedly "value-free" conceptualizations of health and health care.

Boorse's value-free interpretation of the concept of health

The best known proponent of a value-free interpretation of health has been Christopher Boorse. Boorse says that the majority of clinicians and philosophers are "entirely mistaken" in maintaining that "health is an essentially evaluative notion" (1976, 49). This mistake, Boorse says, "rests on a confusion between the theoretical and practical senses of 'health', or in other words, between disease and illness" (Ibid.). Brown describes Boorse's position as follows:

> On Boorse's account, then, a disease is "a type of internal state which is either an impairment of normal functional ability, i.e., a reduction of one or more functional abilities below typical efficiency or a limitation on functional ability caused by environmental agents (Boorse 1977, 567; cited in Brown 1985, 313-314).

Englehardt cashes out Boorse's "biostatistical notion of health" (Nordenfeldt's term) in terms of four key concepts (Nordenfeldt 1987, 16):

> 1. The *reference class* is a natural class of organisms of uniform functional design, an age group of a sex of a species.
> 2. A *normal function* of a part or process within members of the reference class is a statistically typical contribution by it to their individual survival and reproduction.
> 3. A *disease* is a type of internal state which is either an impairment of normal functional ability, i.e., a reduction of one or more functional abilities below typical efficiency, or a limitation on functional ability caused by environmental agents.
> 4. *Health* is the absence of disease.

In this account of health as the absence of disease, two terms, *function* and *statistical normality*, require further explanation. Physiological functions are physical processes that tend toward certain goals, where "goals" are understood as other traits or processes of the organism. Boorse says that "a function in the biologist's sense is nothing but a standard causal contribution to a goal actually pursued by an organism" (Boorse 1976, 57). Biological organisms are conceived in terms of a hierarchy of physiological functions, ultimately culminating in species-typical goals of survival and reproduction (Boorse 1976, 57). Statistical normalities define the normal natural functioning of a species, i.e. the hierarchy of processes and goals that Boorse labels as "*the species design*" (Brown 1985, 313, my italics). Given species design, statistical normalities can be used to define typical functioning as a range of efficiency levels within a selected reference group (say, women over the age of 65). Boorse's main qualification of this essentially statistical approach to defining health and disease is in terms of "limitations on functional ability caused by environmental agents". This qualification lets Boorse account for "nearly universal diseases", such as tooth decay or athereosclerosis, which are statistically normal over the course of the reference group's life span.

Boorse then treats *disease* as a *non-normative, purely empirical, theoretical concept* that applies to both human and non-human organisms. The implication is, as Gordon argues, that "nature" is autonomous – to be distinguished "from the 'supernatural', from human consciousness, from 'culture', 'society', 'morality', 'psychology', and particular time and space" (Gordon 1988, 23). Accordingly, Gordon says,

> Biomedical practitioners approach sickness as a natural phenomenon, legitimize and develop their knowledge using a naturalist method (scientific rationality) and see themselves as practising on nature's human representative – the human body. (Gordon 1988, 24)

In this naturalizing approach, I would suggest, there is also *a divorce* between "cure" and "care", in which cure is treated as an objective, scientific, and naturalistic endeavour and care as a normatively laden and culturally situated enterprise. Cure consists in the achievement of the biological state of normalcy. In practice care is subordinated to the achievement of cure. This is shown in the subordinate place of palliative medicine in the hierarchy of traditional biomedicine where surgery and other acute care areas are ranked highly. The cure–care distinction suggests one way of interpreting Anderson and Reimer Kirkham's finding of "holism" amongst those they interviewed as involving a desire to reintegrate the opposites in question, particularly those of "cure" and "care", as well as "mind" and "body" (Anderson and Reimer Kirkham, chapter 4). The promise of overcoming these divisions is perhaps part of the appeal of alternative medicine and a likely reason for the distrust of biomedicine in various parts of the Canadian population.[3]

Boorse says that physiological health or the absence of disease can be described as *normally desirable* in that most people want (a) the goals of physiological health, such as survival and reproduction, and (b) the attendant activities, to wit, sex and eating (Boorse 1976, 60). However, the actual desirability of health and the undesirability of disease are contingent on personal preferences and life circumstances. For example, sexually mature individuals may well find it desirable to be infertile at times, and youths facing conscription may be happy to find they have flat feet, even though both infertility and flat feet are deviations from species normality and, in Boorse's disease related sense, "unhealthy".

This sets the stage for Boorse's distinction between "disease" and "illness". Unlike *disease* which he treats as a purely empirical or scientific concept, *Boorse defines illness* as an inherently normative concept. Illnesses "are merely a subclass of diseases, namely, those diseases that have certain normative features reflected in the institutions of medical practice" (Boorse 1976, 56).[4] Thus, he offers this definition:

> A disease is an illness only if it is serious enough to be incapacitating, and therefore is (i) *undesirable to its bearer*, (ii) *a title to special treatment*, and (iii) *a valid excuse for normally criticizable behaviour* (Boorse 1976, 61, my emphasis).

Boorse uses the disease–illness distinction to mark a distinction between medical *practice*, which deals with illness, and medical *science*, which deals with disease.

Culture, illness, and disease

Where does culture enter Boorse's conceptualization of illness and disease?[5] Culture would presumably be relevant to Boorse's notion of illness insofar as it is reflected in its three defining conditions. Thus, with regard to (i), if most members of culture A regarded the incapacitating disease as undesirable and members of most other cultures (B through Z) did not, then presumably culture would be salient in developing an empirical understanding of the role that illness plays in culture A (descriptive ethics) and in forming relevant ethical judgements about what is desirable in culture A (normative ethics).[6] With regard to (ii) and (iii), Boorse's account would also allow and invite culturally specific explanations of patterns of illness. Thus in culture A, particular diseases could well connect to (ii) entitlements to special treatment and (iii) be an excuse for normally criticizable actions, whereas in cultures B, C, and D, the disease might go unmarked and unnoticed on both the entitlement and responsibility dimensions.

With regard to Boorse's conceptualization of disease in terms of a biostatistical or physiological conception of health, it seems unlikely that culture would be regarded as having much significance except in one respect. This occurs with respect to Boorse's use of reference classes to identify some types of diseases, e.g. diseases of women, men, and neonates. Presumably some reference classes would be linked to particular cultures via linking notions like occupation, race, religion, ethnicity, and presumably genetics (insofar as we reconstruct notions of family, ethnicity, and race on a genetic basis).[7]

Nonetheless the main effect of Boorse's disease based analysis of health would be to encourage those in "practical medicine" (Boorse's term) towards non-cultural, that is culturally decontextualized, understandings of diseases and even most illnesses. This is because the conception of physiological normality that is central to Boorse's analysis of health rests on the assumption that there are generic human preference patterns with regard to most diseases. That is, most illnesses are likely to be common across cultures with differences only at the margins. Thus a major effect of Boorse's disease–illness distinction would be to reinforce the idea of medicine and health care as based on a purely biological science that must for the sake of scientific rigour purge itself of reference to context, history, or culture (cf. Gordon 1988).

Anderson and Reimer Kirkham have noted "the implications that the fracturing of disease and illness into separate entities has for the professional division of labour" (Anderson and Reimer Kirkham 1996, 8) in terms of division of what presumably would be described as the "soft" and "unscientific" work of nursing from the "hard" and "scientific" work of doctoring.[8] This suggests a parallel division at the meta-level between those who study disease (biomedical scientists) and those who study illness (social scientists and others engaged in qualitative research).

In response to my criticisms of Boorse's disease–illness division, a defender of Boorse might offer a more positive reading of the disease–illness distinction, namely that the distinction provides at the practical level a useful division of *authority* and at the intellectual level a useful division of *labour*; that it gives health care scientists authority over disease but not over illness. Illness then lies in the realm of morality and politics and not in that of scientific and medical authority. Thus in the illness domain, it could be claimed that people individually as health care recipients (exercising their individual autonomy) and collectively (acting as citizens in the process of democratic decision making) are supreme. Hence, we the people can and should tell health scientists to restrict their work to the purely empirical realm and remain "servants" of patients and society. A parallel argument could be advanced in the intellectual realm, namely that disease is the turf of the hard scientists and illness belongs to those in the "soft" areas of the social sciences and the humanities.

In response I would make three points. First, this putative defence of Boorse is based on a value-laden claim, namely that societies will do better if they divorce control over the treatment and analysis of disease from that of illness. This is itself a controversial claim. Nonetheless, its truth or falsity is quite independent of whether or not anyone can construct a completely value-free notion of disease, health, and health research. Second, a way of testing this claim is to look at societies in which health care providers explicitly take up moral roles. Lock does this in her discussion of the way in which Japanese psychologists deal with children who repeatedly refuse to attend school (Lock 1988b). She says that psychologists see themselves as restoring the traditional moral order prescribed in Confucian thought and not as acting in the "behaviourial" mode of Western psychologists rooted in a value-free conception of biomedicine (Lock 1988b, 406-7). Third, as I argue below, using the disease–illness distinction to mark the boundaries of biomedical and political authority obscures the way in which biomedical authority figures play a political role.[9] It ignores the value-ladenness of the concept of health.

Problems with Boorse's account

I now turn to salient philosophical criticisms of Boorse's biostatistical conception of health and disease.[10] The primary criticism has been that there is no purely empirical or value-free way for Boorse to identify the reference groups that provide the baselines for determining normal species functioning (Brown 1985, 315). Hence a completely naturalistic concept of disease and of cure is not sustainable. This problem of scientifically selecting reference points without resort to ethical norms and values is even more acute when one tries to determine what is the appropriate biological level for determining normal functioning. Thus Nordenfeldt asks why, on Boorse's conception of disease, one should not focus on specific organs rather than the organism as whole, say, on the normal functioning of kidneys rather than that of the whole human organism, e.g. a "healthy kidney" in a "diseased body" (Nordenfeldt 1987, 27). Or one might push the reference point from the individual organism to the species. What is good for the species survival or reproduction need not be beneficial to individual members of the species. For example, high mortality levels may well enhance evolutionary adaptability once reproduction is completed (Englehardt 1982, 74; see also Brown 1985, 316). In other cases Boorse's definition of "disease" has the counterintuitive result that diseases can be described as "a species-typical reaction, i.e. a healthy response to a difficult environment", to wit, "infectious disease … as the species typical reaction to the circumstances of a certain microbial invasion" (Nordenfeldt 1987, 30) or sickle cell anaemia as an adaptation to malaria.

From the perspective of a purely naturalistic science, it also seems arbitrary to focus on survival and reproduction as archetypal ultimate goals. Selecting these as key reference points introduces at least implicitly an evaluative perspective into what was supposed to be a scientific and completely value-free conception of disease and health. Even if it is claimed that survival and reproduction are typical disciplinary perspectives of some of those who study disease and health (e.g. biologists and physiologists), it is reasonable to ask why these disciplinary perspectives should be privileged over others (e.g. those of social scientists and humanists). Once survival and reproduction are introduced as defining goals, it is fair to ask about other ends or goals that humans typically have – e.g. the quest for meaningfulness and community that underlies so many religious (see chapters 2 and 3 above) and non-religious ways of life. This would open the way to thinking of health with reference to the much wider range of ends adopted by human beings in all their diversity rather than limiting it to the admittedly important but narrower ends of survival and reproduction.[11] For example, setting health into the context of the Buddhist conception of *kamma* (chapters 2 and 3) provides a rather different reading of health and health care than would be given in a secularized Western context.

Evaluative conceptions of health

I now turn to conceptions of health and its correlates that are explicitly evaluative. Some of these will reflect Jensen and Allen's view that, "[t]here are no universal norms of health; perceptions vary across individuals and cultures" (cited in Anderson and Reimer Kirkham 1996, 4). Others involve an attempt to construct cross-cultural concepts of health and health care.

In the cross-cultural mode is the well known 1946 World Health Organisation (WHO) definition: "Health is a state of complete physical, mental, and social well-being and not merely the absence of infirmity" (WHO 1946, 48).

The 1946 WHO definition has been criticized as being overexpansive: it makes health tantamount to happiness and not simply an important contribution to it. As well, the definition confers too much authority and expertise on the medical profession (Callahan 1973, 50-51). Contrast this with 1984 WHO definition of health:

> [Health is] the extent to which an individual or group is able, on the one hand to develop aspirations and satisfy needs; and, on the other hand, to change or cope with the environment. Health is therefore seen as a resource for everyday life, not the objective of living; it is seen as a positive concept emphasizing social and personal resources, as well as physical capacities. (WHO European Region 1984, cited in Anderson and Reimer Kirkham 1996, 3)

The 1984 definition usefully restricts the scope of the concept of health, as well as the intellectual and practical authority of health scientists and health providers. As Nordenfeldt notes, health is neither a necessary nor a sufficient condition for happiness; it is, however, connected to happiness or the achievement of important personal goals,

Health is a person's ability, in standard circumstances, to realize his minimal happiness. It is not sufficient for happiness since, if circumstances are not standard, for instance in cases of accident or war, health need not result in happiness. Nor is health necessary for happiness, since the vital goals of an ill but happy person can to a great extent be fulfilled by persons other than the person himself, for instance relatives and others taking care of him. (Nordenfeldt 1987, xv)

Nonetheless my primary concern in this chapter is not with whether these definitions define a distinct area of practice and theory but rather with the implications for cross-cultural health care ethics of treating health and disease as primarily normative concepts. One result is quite clear, namely that health and disease must be understood as ways of labelling wanted or unwanted conditions, not as value-free scientific categories found in nature independent of cultural and social context (Gordon 1988). Englehardt says,

The concept of disease acts not only to describe and explain, but also to enjoin to action. ... It is a normative concept: it says what ought not to be. As such, the concept incorporates criteria of evaluation, designating certain states as desirable and others as not so. It delineates and establishes social roles such as being sick or being a physician. ... The concept is both aesthetic and ethical, suggesting what is beautiful and good. (Englehardt 1975, cited in Brown 1985, 318)

Thus Englehardt describes how masturbation was regarded as a disease in the eighteenth and nineteenth centuries; similarly "drapetomania, the disease causing slaves to run away" was regarded as disease in the U.S. south. (Englehardt 1974, 59, 62). In our times, alcoholism, drug addiction, and smoking could be added to the list. Thomas Szasz is well known for his arguments concerning "the myth of mental illness" as a way of labelling as "deviant" socially unwanted behaviours (Szasz 1960).[12]

Now one upshot of the evaluative conceptualization is that it may usefully focus attention on moral and political reform rather than on a medicalized abnormality, e.g. getting rid of slavery rather than finding a cure for drapetomania. In other cases, it could lead in the opposite direction – to the political judgement that the state of affairs in question (e.g. allowing smoking in public buildings) is indeed undesirable. In either case, it is worth asking if the normative perspective is culture specific or if it has trans-cultural appeal. For other conditions the disabling or disagreeable aspects of the condition seem to apply quite generally; extreme fatigue, pain, and disablement might be transculturally regarded as salient features of psychophysiological states that are candidates for being counted amongst the negative correlates of health. (Though even here it should be noted that sleep deprivation has been used to induce states in which spiritual insight can be encouraged.) But it is essential to understand that the meaning and significance of health and its negative correlates including disease, disability, incapacity, and even dying (as in Stephenson's account of death amongst the Hutterites) can vary significantly from one context to another (Stephenson 1983). In Part I, my colleagues provide ample illustrations of these notions in a wide variety of contexts including Chinese, Buddhist, and in Part III, Native Canadian.

Wants, needs, and health

I now want to consider an objection to the approach I have taken in this chapter. The objection is that the adoption of an evaluative reading of health, disease, and illness (and the correlative rejection of "biomedical imperialism") seems to leave health care providers and recipients, especially in cross-cultural interactions, in a moral vacuum.[13] "This", my imagined objector might contend, "is because an evaluative notion of health simply turns health into an object of personal preferences or wants. What a healthy state is becomes a variable depending on the preferences of the individuals or groups in question. The very meanings of health, disease, and illness must be linked to individual and collective evaluations. While this approach yields an evaluative notion of health that is culturally specific, it fails to provide goals that other than accidentally have cross-cultural significance. We are left then with no inter-culturally compelling reading of the meaning and significance of health and health care."

In response, I want to suggest another way of construing health and health care so that we can find a basis for constructing cross-culturally compelling health care agendas.[14] My way of doing this is through an examination of needs based readings of the notion of health. These have been advanced by a number of philosophers, including Norman Daniels in his important 1985 book, *Just Health Care*. Daniels carefully crafted a Rawlsian argument for the state's provision of health care. From a more philosophy of science perspective, Lennart Nordenfeldt has presented an action–theoretic approach to the nature of health that is essentially based on the idea of needs. I will however focus on Caroline Whitbeck's account of disease and health in terms of capabilities because it offers a useful way of thinking about health in the context of ways of life. Whitbeck offers this reading of the concept of disease:

> The definition of *disease* that I have offered is that diseases are, first of all, psychophysiological processes; second, they compromise the ability to do what people commonly want and expect to be able to do; third, they are not necessary in order to do what people commonly want to be able to do; fourth, they are either statistically abnormal in those at risk or there is some other basis for a reasonable hope of finding means to effectively treat or prevent them. (Whitbeck 1981, 20)

It is worth looking at the four criteria in turn. The first locates disease in the category of physiological and psychological processes. The second helps to identify the basis for our "interest in being able to do something about" diseases; for diseases compromise "what people commonly want and expect to be able to do". This offers a helpful way of thinking about traditional and alternative (revealingly described in French as *les médicines douces* or "soft" medicines). Wants have to be set in life contexts, and this includes cultural, religious, political, moral, and other beliefs and commitments that people happen to have. The third criterion, that the condition in question is "not necessary in order to do what people want to be able to do", is relevant for eliminating from the category of diseases such conditions as a normal pregnancy, which despite its discomforts and interferences with normal functioning may well be highly desired. The fourth criterion – that the disease is "statistically abnormal in those at risk or there is some other basis for a reasonable hope of finding means to effectively treat or prevent" the condition – offers an opportunity for transcultural dialogue about health and disease without however ignoring cultural context. That is, it still is essential to define the disease relative to what the people in question "commonly want or expect to be able to do" within the context of their ways of life.

Whitbeck contextualizes her concept of disease:

> According to these criteria, what qualifies as a disease is relative to a societal context insofar as what people are understood as wanting to do is relative to societal context.[15]

So on Whitbeck's account societal context is essential to conceptualizing diseases as interferences in what people want to do. My reading of this is that diseases have social meanings and interpretations, that is individual understandings of "disease" have to be socially contextualized.

In many cases, the ways of life and normal opportunities will be specific to particular cultures.[16] In other cases there will be significant cross-cultural similarities. For example, the modernizing forces of scientific biomedicine have had beneficial effects in some regards (e.g. the elimination of malaria in tropical areas), yet in other cases the effects have been harmful. Nestlé's much condemned marketing of infant formula as the modern scientific way to raise children is a case in point (Velasquez 1983, 304-312).[17] Let me suggest here that the worldwide campaign against Nestlé is an instance of creating a cross-culturally compelling shared agenda on health care.

Whitbeck defines health as follows:

> Health is a person's psychophysiological capacity to act or respond appropriately (in a way that is supportive of the person's goals, projects, and aspirations) in a wide variety of situations. Health encompasses certain significant components: among them, maintaining physical fitness, having a

generally realistic view of situations, and having the ability to discharge
negative feelings. (Whitbeck 1981, 24)[18]

It is important to understand that this concept of health locates individuals
in their communities. Thus Whitbeck says,

> To assess people's health, one must take into account their capabilities, and
> not merely their biological capacities. Therefore, the notion of health or
> wholeness is closely associated with the ability to act to achieve one's
> purposes, and with *the ability to live as a member of a human community.*
> (Whitbeck 1981, 21, my emphasis)

While analytically Whitbeck's notion of health refers both to individuals and
communities, the reality is that individuals lead their lives as members of
particular human communities. Health assessment then has to focus on
individuals in specific communities. This has implications for a conception
of health that is holistic in seeing health in social context and not simply as a
characteristic of asocial individuals conceived as normally functioning
biological units.

Setting shared agendas

Thus far in this chapter I have introduced and criticized value-free
conceptions of health; next I presented Whitbeck's analysis of health and its
negative correlates as an example of a useful evaluative analysis of these
concepts. It is fair to ask how far this takes us towards conceptions of health
and health care that are both culturally sensitive and morally responsive to
the need to establish shared social agendas in the face of cultural diversity.
This need is pressing in multicultural societies like Canada. But it is also
important in much more culturally and religiously homogeneous societies
like Thailand. Even Thailand has its minority populations. Even more
pressing for Thailand is the rapid process of modernization that it and its
neighbours in Southeast Asia are undergoing. That is, cultures in change
face major problems of cultural diversity between the old and the new, the
traditional and the modern. Moreover cultural diversity and change goes
beyond borders. Thus biomedicine with its Western origins has affected
Thailand and many other countries. At the same time, traditional medicines
(e.g. Chinese herbal medicines) have a major impact on Western views of
health and health care. While we do not live in a world without borders
(consider the profound differences between health care delivery in Canada
and the United States), borders do not stop the flow of ideas or economic
and political influences. Consider the pervasive effects of multinational
pharmaceutical companies in determining national health policies, all the
way from setting health care research agendas to the training of medical
practitioners.

So what I have been seeking are evaluative conceptions of health, disease, and the like (e.g. health care and cure) that are pluralistic enough to be responsive to morally significant cultural and religious differences but not so relativistic as to make impossible agreement and action on social agendas that are responsive to an important range of human needs. I introduced Whitbeck's account of health and disease because I think it is at least *structurally* the right sort of account. In her account diseases are presented as obstacles to "what people commonly want to be able to do" (Whitbeck 1981, 20). Conceptualizing health as a capacity "to act or respond appropriately (in a way that is supportive of the person's goals, projects, and aspirations) in a wide variety of situations" provides enough structural commonalties for people with very diverse goals, projects, and aspirations to work together, that is to negotiate shared moral and political agendas around the achievement of health and the provision of health care.

To be clear about this, let me distinguish the sort of account I favour – where health is a good and disease, handicap, etc. are evils – from Norman Daniels's needs based account of health. Following Braybrooke, Daniels describes needs as objectively ascribable and objectively important (Braybrooke 1987; Daniels 1985, 25).[19] Daniels wants both features to build an account of justice in health care that is to a considerable extent independent of variances in individual preferences.[20] The fulfilment of needs is something that any rational or prudent individual will want regardless of her particular life plans. That is, regardless of life plan, individuals will want what Rawls calls "primary goods" (Rawls 1971, 92). The primary social goods (the sorts of goods that a society can distribute to its members) are "rights and liberties, opportunities and powers, income and wealth". Primary natural goods include "health and vigour, intelligence and imagination (Rawls 1971, 62)." Daniels makes the substantive claim that health care is a primary social good. Specifically with respect to health care needs, Daniels takes as his main reference point Boorse's "species-typical normal functioning" (Daniels 1985, 26). What is critical for Daniels is that health care needs be "*uncontroversial* and *ascertainable through publicly acceptable methods,* such as biomedical sciences" (Daniels 1985, 30).[21]

Daniels's concern with health care is its contribution to maintaining or restoring "a normal opportunity range" for individuals. Relevant to our purposes, normal opportunity ranges are determined in relation to social context:

> The *normal opportunity range* for a given society is the array of life-plans reasonable people in it are likely to construct for themselves. The normal range is thus dependent on key features of a society – its stage of historical development, its level of material wealth and technological development, and even important cultural facts about it. This is one way in which the notion of normal opportunity range is socially relative. (Daniels 1985, 33)

Later Daniels says that because normal opportunities are "defined by reference to particular societies, the same disease in two societies may impair opportunity differently and so have its importance assessed differently" (Daniels 1985, 34). In this connection, he mentions the importance dyslexia has in a literate, as opposed to a pre-literate, society.[22]

In Daniels's account, with respect to health care needs all of us humans are both *structurally* and *substantively* the same. Structurally health is primary or basic in the sense of being basically desirable in all rational life plans.[23] Substantively all of us humans are alike in the sense of health being the same or identical good in each person's life plan; hence we have the same basic health care needs. So we are *structurally* alike in that health (in both the absence of disease sense and the positive state sense) is normally quite important to each of us (e.g. whether or not we are Christian or non-Christian, Buddhist or non-Buddhist, a follower of traditional Chinese medicine or scientific biomedicine). And we are substantively alike in that the goods we seek in being healthy and the evils we fear in being diseased, handicapped, or impaired are substantively the same regardless of our culture, religion, etc. So cultural, religious, and social understandings of health and disease appear in this account as "add-ons" to a common core of objectively determinable and rationally desirable conditions. To use a distinction from medieval philosophy, Daniels offers a univocal account of health as a good. The structural account I favour treats these as analogous goods.

I believe that in his univocal account of health care needs Daniels concedes too much to the neutrality and authority of biomedical sciences. I would suggest that a culturally sensitive and sociologically sophisticated bioethics can meet this challenge better than abstract and culturally unsituated "biomedical sciences". It is hard to see in Daniels's account how universalistic, naturalizing biomedical sciences can make the appropriate references to "social roles" and "normal opportunity ranges" available in diverse societies without entering the area of moral and political choice. Moreover in trying to arrive at morally justifiable judgments about the provision of health care, it will be essential to distinguish between actual and desirable normal opportunity ranges.

Daniels would try to make this distinction by hypothesizing a Rawlsian "original position" from which to consider health care needs. Behind the veil of ignorance in the original position no one knows their specific identity (gender, status, talents, abilities, disabilities, etc.); hence, everyone would know that they will likely have some health care needs but not which health care needs are specifically theirs. Following Rawls, Daniels thinks that people in such a position would imagine themselves potentially in the situation of the worst-off members of society and make social arrangements accordingly. To put this another way, behind the veil of ignorance in the original position everyone can see that they will be culturally situated but no one knows what their particular culture will be. Daniels wants to build his normative account of just health care on a thin account of the goods of health and the evils of its negative correlates.[24]

My suggestion is to remain rooted in thick accounts of the goods of health and the evils of its opposite numbers. In health care provision, it is important for providers to be aware that diseases like cancer or AIDS or particular mental or physical disabilities or handicaps can have different meanings for one health care consumer (e.g. a Thai Buddhist) than another (e.g. a secular Canadian). To be sure, both see the conditions in question as (perhaps in quite different ways) disabling them and thus standing in the way of what they want to do. But substantively the goods and evils are not the same in both lives – seeing a disease in the context of *kamma* is different from seeing it as purely physiological process (Ratanakul, chapter 2).

It then becomes crucial for health care providers to be aware of their own "cultural perspectives" on the goods and evils in question – whether these be cultures in the traditional sense or the professional cultures of physicians, nurses, etc. Thus a Western psychiatrist treating a Cambodian refugee in Canada for depression needs to be aware not only of her patient's world-view, but also of her own cultural perspectives as a professional psychiatrist (Stephenson, chapter 5).

Cure, care, culture, and community

Thus far, the focus of my remarks has been on the place of culture in understanding health and health care. I have argued against the idea that these are value-free concepts and claimed that treating them as value free conceals significant normative commitments. I have also said that "curing" like "caring" has to be located in particular cultures. Curing and caring involve social relations. They also involve the formal and informal organization of societal practices and institutions and thus have to do with the construction and uses of power and authority in societies.

In arguing that "health is not a purely biological concept", Nordenfeldt says that the concept of health should be understood as containing

> an essential reference to an environment involving a society. Thus, the clarification of the discourse on health cannot be made merely by improving our biological or broadly medical conceptual apparatus. As noted ... there must be a standing request to each society to specify the vital goals to be adopted in a particular society. These requests are profound and entail a major demand on the social politics of the governing bodies in society. (Nordenfeldt 1987, 129)

To address health care needs adequately, there needs to be a discussion in each society or community of "vital goals" or of what Daniels describes as "the normal opportunity range for that society ... (that is) the array of life-plans reasonable people in it are likely to construct for themselves" (Daniels 1985, 20). This involves reflection on the diverse cultural, religious, etc. meanings of "health" and "health care" that members of the society have. In some societies, like Thailand, this will involve reflection on values rooted in a common but rapidly changing culture. In a multicultural society like Canada, there needs to be a dialogue amongst people of diverse and changing cultures – the fair negotiation in other words of a shared social agenda for health care.

I would suggest then that in order to adequately address the question of "health as a social responsibility", it is essential to move from consideration of just three Cs of *cure, care,* and *culture* to a fourth C, *community.* The essential ethical question then is about the kind of community that best reflects a society's moral sensibilities. Is it an inclusive community or one that excludes and marginalizes on the basis of gender, race, and class? Is it a community in which solidarity is prized or is it one that devalues solidarity to serve only the interests of a select few? Locating questions of cure and care in cultural context takes us then to the crucial ethical questions around various communities' collective provision for meeting significant health care needs.

Notes

1. I wish to give credit to my colleagues – particularly Burgess, Anderson, and Stephenson – for helping me come to grips with what I now see as the strongly platonizing tendencies of analytic philosophy and much of contemporary moral philosophy in my own work.

2. Meta-ethics or theoretical ethics is the part of ethics that deals with the meaning of ethical terms and their justification.

3. This distrust was manifest in the general discussion following a symposium in May 1996 on alternative health care approaches sponsored by the Vancouver Multicultural Society. Over two hundred people attended the symposium. The symposium was to mark the establishment of the Tzu Chi Institute at Vancouver Hospital and Health Science Centre. The Tzu Chi Institute is dedicated to research on alternative medicine and is sponsored by a Buddhist society based in Taiwan. I was one of the keynote speakers at this event.

4. Kleinman makes a similar distinction: "Disease refers to a malfunctioning of biological and/or psychological processes, while the term illness refers to the psychosocial experience and meaning of perceived disease. Illness includes secondary personal and social responses to a primary malfunctioning (disease) in the individual's physiological status (or both)" (Kleinman 1980, 72).

5. My reading of "culture" follows Stephenson's idea of "culture as a broad and deep influence on all human behaviour which is simultaneously personal and social", including of course those doing ethics or, for that matter, sociology (Stephenson 1985, 2).

6. *Normative ethics* is the branch of ethics concerned not so much with studying or theorizing about but with actually making normative judgments in morals and values; that is making judgments about actions, persons, and their character, using a moral and value vocabulary. As ethics (contrasted with naive morality) it makes use of, or is informed by, reflection on descriptive and theoretical ethics.

Descriptive ethics is the part of ethics that describes the morals and values of individuals or groups, as these morals and values are shown in customs, practices, traditions, and ideologies. Based on the work of anthropologists, sociologists, and other social scientists, as well as the direct study of texts and the testimony of informants, it attempts to interpret and structure practices and the ways in which one might attempt to ground or justify them. (McDonald et al. 1992, i, iii).

7. Brown doubts that within his theory Boorse can consistently allow such reference classes; nonetheless Boorse claims that his theory does allow these (Brown 1985, 315). Later I discuss this with regard to Nordenfeldt's idea of society as a "background" for health care activities.

8. However, as noted above, Boorse thinks that most doctors are on the "soft" or "practice" side of medicine.

9. Thus the hard data of health science is used to discount the soft data of politics and morality in such key areas as cost–benefit analysis and risk management.

10. These philosophical criticisms identify problems *internal* to Boorse's account. These internal criticisms should be distinguished from the *external* criticisms of sociologists, anthropologists, and others (such as Lock, Gordon, Stephenson, and Englehardt) of the very idea of constructing a completely acultural, naturalistic discourse of biomedicine.

11. It is not my intention here to discuss whether survival and reproduction could be meaningful ends in themselves, that is, valued for their own sake and not as means to more ultimate ends.

12. It should be noted that a main reason that Szasz thinks mental illness is a myth is that the only non-mythical diseases in these categories are "diseases of the brain". That is, Szasz buys into the value-free conception of disease (Szasz 1960, 76-77).

13. By "biomedical imperialism" I mean the view that there is an authoritative, value-free reading of health, disease, and related concepts that is the special province of health scientists.

14. See McDonald (1995) for an exploration of the idea of constructing common moral agendas.

15. Whitbeck does go on to say: "Statistical abnormality in those at risk (world-wide) however is *independent* of societal context. Therefore, a psychophysiological process may qualify as a disease even if a society fails to *recognise* its presence because of its near ubiquity of those at risk in that society (Whitbeck 1981, 20).

16. King's 1954 definition is similar: "Disease is the aggregate of those conditions which, judged by the prevailing culture, are deemed painful, or disabling, and which, at the same time deviate from either the statistical norm or from some other idealised status" (Lester King 1954, cited in Brown 1985, 318).

17. Nestlé marketed the formula in countries where it was virtually impossible for most of the population to get clean water to mix with the powdered formula. They even dressed salespeople as "nurses" to promote the formula. The net effect was that very poor people stopped breast feeding and used scarce resources to buy the formula – a formula that was promoted on billboards as representing the scientific way to feed children. The WHO and numerous health organisations condemned Nestlé's actions.

I am not suggesting that scientific authorities supported Nestlé's marketing efforts.

However, Nestlé was able to use the veneer of scientific medicine to market a product that was, under the conditions offered, exceptionally harmful.

18. Compare this to Nordenfeldt's definition of health: "*A* is in health if, and only if, *A* has the ability, given standard circumstances, to realise his vital goals, i.e. the set of goals which are necessary and together sufficient for his minimal happiness" (Nordenfeldt 1987, 90). There is a connection here between Whitbeck's conception of health and Freeman and Conrad's discussions of personal responsibility for health (Anderson and Reimer Kirkham 1996, 14-15).

19. Braybrooke develops a "List of matters of need" based on an examination of various schedules of needs developed by a variety of scholars. Braybrooke's list has twelve items. The first six centre on physiological functioning: "(1) the need to have a life-supporting relation to the environment, (2) the need for food and water, (3) the need to excrete, (4) the need for exercise, (5) the need for periodic rest, including sleep, and (6) the need (beyond what is covered under the preceding) for whatever is indispensable to preserving the body intact in important respects." The final six have to do with "functioning as a social being": "(7) the need for companionship, (8) the need for education, (9) the need for social acceptance and recognition, (10) the need for sexual activity, (11) the need to be free from harassment, including not being continually frightened, and (12) the need for recreation" (Braybrooke 1987, 36)

20. The obvious problems is to avoid, on the one hand, creating a right to health care that even the wealthiest societies would be unable to satisfy while, on the other hand, being so parsimonious with the right that the needs of many (particularly the worst-off) are unaddressed.

21. He goes on to say that "[i]t will not matter if what counts as a disease is relative to some features of social roles in a given society, and thus to some normative judgements, provided the core of the notion of species normal functioning is left intact". Daniels hopes that his account of health care needs will allow him to avoid the argument over whether health is a descriptive or an evaluative concept (30). It is worth noting that Daniels has a fairly wide conception of health care needs including: (1) adequate nutrition and shelter; (2) sanitary, safe, unpolluted living and working conditions; (3) exercise, rest, and some features of life-style; (4) preventive, curative, and rehabilitative personal medical services; and (5) non-medical personal and social support services (32).

22. Another example given by Daniels is also relevant here, namely, in regard to health insurance payments for plastic surgery. He cites the controversy in Massachusetts when Blue Cross refused to pay for reconstructive plastic surgery following mastectomies. Daniels suggests that such refusal was unfair because the surgery can be seen as necessary for restoring a normal opportunity range to the women in question (Daniels 1985, 31). After public controversy, Blue Cross reversed its policy.

23. Rawls says, "a person's good is determined by what is for him the most rational long-term plan given reasonably favourable circumstances" (Rawls 1971, 92-93). A life-plan is rational in the sense that it permits "the harmonious satisfaction of (a person's) interests", and it is "arrived at by rejecting other plans that are either less likely to succeed or do not provide for such an inclusive attainment of aims" (Rawls 1971, 93).

24. "Thin" and "thick" are terms introduced by Rawls to describe accounts of the good from behind the veil of ignorance and as seen when the veil is lifted.

References

Anderson, Joan M. and Sheryl Reimer Kirkham. 1996. Health and illness. Unpublished paper.

Boorse, Christopher. 1975. On the distinction between disease and illness. *Philosophy and Public Affairs* 5, 1 (Fall): 49-68.

Braybrooke, David. 1987. *Meeting needs*. Princeton, NJ: Princeton University Press.

Burgess, Michael and Patricia Rodney. 1995. Western ethical theory and concepts: evolution and opportunities for cross-cultural health care ethics. Ms.

Callahan, Daniel. 1973. The WHO Definition of health. *The Hastings Center Report*, 1:3 (1973). Reprinted in *Readings in biomedical ethics: a Canadian focus*. Eike-Henner W. Kluge, ed., pp. 6-16.

Coward, Harold. 1995. Participation in health care decision-making on issues surrounding life and death in Hinduism and Buddhism. Unpublished paper.

Daniels, Norman. 1985. *Just health care*. Cambridge: Cambridge U.P.

Englehardt, Tristram. 1976. Human well-being and medicine: some basic value-judgements in biomedical science. In *Science, ethics, and medicine*, ed. H. T. Englehardt and D. Callahan. Institute of Society, Ethics and the Life Sciences.

———. 1974. The disease of masturbation: values and the concept of disease. *Bulletin of the History of Medicine,* Vol. 48, No. 2 (Summer): 234-248. Reprinted in *Contemporary issues in bioethics*, second edition, 1982, ed. Tom Beauchamp and LeRoy Walters, 59-63. Belmont CA: Wadsworth Publishing, pp. .

———. 1982. The roles of values in the discovery of illnesses, diseases, and disorders. *Contemporary issues in bioethics*, second edition, ed. Tom Beauchamp and LeRoy Walters, 73-75. Belmont CA: Wadsworth Publishing.

Feinberg, Joel. 1970. *Doing and deserving: Essays in the theory of responsibility*. Princeton: Princeton U.P.

———. Crime, clutchability, and individuated treatment. In: *Doing and deserving*. Princeton: Princeton U.P., pp. 252-271.

Flew, Anthony. 1973. *Crime or disease?* London: Macmillan.

Gauthier, David. 1976. The social contract as ideology. *Philosophy and Public Affairs* 6, 2.

Gordon, Deborah R. 1988. Tenacious assumptions in western medicine. In *Biomedicine examined*, ed. M. Lock and D. R. Gordon, 19-56. Dordrecht: Kluwer Publishing.

Guttmacher, Sally. 1979. Whole in body, mind, and spirit: Holistic health and the limits of medicine. *Hastings Center Report* 9 (April): 15-18, 20-21.

Kato, Hisatake. 1986.What Is bioethics? Tokyo: Mirai-Sya.

Kleinman, Arthur. 1980. *Patients and healers in the context of culture: An explanation of the borderland between anthropology, medicine, and psychiatry.* Berkeley, CA: University of California Press.

Lock, Margaret. 1988a. Introduction. In *Biomedicine examined*, ed. M. Lock and D. R. Gordon, 3-16. Dordrecht: Kluwer Publishing.

Lock, Margaret. 1988b. A nation at risk: Interpretations of school refusal in Japan. In *Biomedicine examined*, ed. M. Lock and D. R. Gordon, 377-414. Dordrecht: Kluwer Publishing.

McDonald, Michael, J. T. Stevenson, and Wesley Cragg. 1992. *Finding a balance of values: An ethical assessment of Ontario Hydro's demand/supply plan. report to the Aboriginal research coalition of Ontario.* Filed before the Ontario Environmental Assessment Board.

McDonald, Michael. 1995."Prescriptions from religious and secular ethics for breaking the impoverishment/environmental degradation cycle. In *Consumption and the Environment: Religious and secular perspectives*, ed. Harold Coward, 195-216. Albany NY: State University of New York Press.

Nickel, James. 1987. *Making sense of human rights: Philosophical reflections on the Universal Declaration of Human Rights*. Berkeley, CA: University of California Press.

Nordenfeldt, Lennart. 1987. On the nature of health: An action–theoretic approach. Dordrecht: D. Reidel. Reprinted in *Contemporary issues in bioethics*, ed. Tom Beauchamp and LeRoy Walters, 54-59.Belmont CA: Wadsworth Publishing, .

Rawls, John. 1971. *A theory of justice*. Cambridge, MA: Harvard University Press.

Shue, Henry. 1980. *Basic rights*. Princeton: Princeton, UP.

Stephenson, Peter. 1983. "He died too quick!": The process of dying in a Hutterian colony. *Omega*, 14(2) pp. 127-134.

———. 1995. Expanding and refining notions of culture for an inter-cultural ethics in medicine. Ms.

Szasz, Thomas. 1986. The myth of mental illness. *The American Psychologist.* Reprinted in *Contemporary issues in bioethics*, second edition, ed. Tom Beauchamp and LeRoy Walters, 263-9. Belmont CA: Wadsworth Publishing, pp. .

Taylor, Charles. 1995. Two theories of modernity." *Hastings Center Report* 25, 2 (March-April), pp. 24-32.

Whitbeck, Caroline. 1981. A theory of health. In *Concepts of health and disease: interdisciplinary perspectives*, ed. A. I. Caplan, H. T. Englehardt, and J. J. McCartney, . Reading, 611-626. MA: Addison-Wellesley Publishing. Reprinted in *Readings in biomedical ethics: A Canadian focus*, ed. Eike-Henner W. Kluge, 16-29.

World Health Organisation. 1946. Preamble to the Constitution of the World Health Organisation. Reprinted in *Contemporary issues in bioethics*, second edition, Tom Beauchamp and LeRoy Walters, 48. Belmont CA: Wadsworth Publishing, p. 48.

Part I, Conclusion

Harold Coward

The above chapters have presented a conceptual analysis of the ways in which "culture", "health", and "illness" may be understood as establishing a basic foundation for cross-cultural health care ethics. After being introduced to the quite different basic assumptions underlying these concepts in Thai Buddhist and Chinese thought, we were sensitized to the multiple meanings of health provided by various social contexts – including the cultural context of biomedicine itself. Anderson and Reimer Kirkham's feminist and post-colonial analysis revealed the powerful influence of race, gender, and class relations upon health and health care in various historical and cultural contexts. These influences were poignantly illustrated in the voices of their community respondents – for example in the need to address poverty, sexism, and the exploitation of the underclasses, when the allocation of resources between health care and the social conditions needed for health is discussed as an ethical issue. Stephenson continued this critique by examining the different assumptions that lie behind the uses of the term "culture" and the implications for ethics. Stephenson demonstrated that biomedicine falsely assumes that it is a privileged or neutral site where culture does not play a role. He calls for (and attempts to provide) an expanded self-awareness on the part of practitioners and researchers that biomedical science is itself a culture.

McDonald concluded Part I by further testing this thesis. He conducted a careful philosophical analysis of Boorse's argument that there can be a value-free and culture-neutral concept of health and medicine. Finding Boorse's argument flawed in key respects, McDonald then showed how one could develop a philosophical basis that would respect fundamental cultural and religious differences and yet allow for shared values of the sort needed for the development of cross-cultural health care ethics. In line with the other authors in Part I, McDonald warns against the dangers, for ethics, of overemphasizing the needs and rights of individuals at the expense of collective identities and minority communities. Here we are taken back to the ethics of the Chinese and Buddhist perspectives in which not only other human individuals and groups but also our respectful relationship with the natural environment must be considered in order for health to be realized.

By dealing with the major conceptual questions, Part I sets the stage for our examination of three culturally contextualized examples of health care ethics in Part II, before we move on to applied ethical examples in health care delivery (Part III) and policy issues (Part IV).

Part II

Culture and Health Care Ethics

Part II, Introduction

Barry Hoffmaster

As people from diverse cultural and ethnic backgrounds mingle and interact more and more, opportunities for conflict among their beliefs, values, and ways of life proliferate. One emotion-laden example is the use of corporal punishment in child rearing. A reporter observes: "At a time when immigrants make up nearly twenty percent of the Canadian population, one of the biggest cultural confrontations between ethnic minority communities and mainstream culture is about where spanking ends and child abuse begins."[1] Immigrants to this country who were subjected to stern discipline and sometimes spanked or whacked with a stick when they misbehaved and who are now parents themselves can regard the Canadian approach to child rearing as too liberal and too permissive. For many Canadians however corporal punishment is intolerable, not only because it is ineffective but because it teaches children to solve problems by resorting to violence.

How should this conflict between minority and mainstream cultures be handled? Should parents who belong to cultures in which corporal punishment is approved and encouraged be allowed to use it on their children or should they be required to conform to the Canadian way? If respect for cultural diversity is the proper response, what are the limits of this tolerance or cultural sensitivity? If, on the contrary, deference to the views of the majority may legitimately be demanded, what justifies this "cultural imperialism"?

Health care is also rife with cultural differences and potential for conflicts. The most intimate events of our lives – reproduction, birth, death – draw people into the health care system and expose their most fundamental attitudes, values, and beliefs. More generally, concepts of health and disease and expectations about how those who are ill or suffering should behave are suffused with assumptions and values that reflect culturally distinctive views of the nature of persons and their relationships with others, with the world, and with a transcendent order. Health care ethics now faces the increasingly important challenge of figuring out how conflicts that can be deeply embedded in different cultural and religious understandings of life and the world should be handled.

Obviously that is not an easy task. The aim of Part II is to provide some background in terms of how the moral and policy issues raised in the following chapters can be addressed. Buddhist and Chinese approaches to health care ethics relating to the boundary conditions of birth and death are reviewed, along with the secular health care ethics that has evolved in North America over the last several decades. The concluding section then outlines the general questions that need to be asked in order to understand cultural conflicts in health care ethics. As with the other parts of this book, the dialogue between cultures and religions over health care ethics is focused on Buddhist and Chinese traditions as examples but not as exhaustive of the field of study.

Note

1. I. Vincent, "Rather spank than spoil", *Globe and Mail*, 24 April 1996, A1, A10.

Chapter 7
Buddhist Health Care Ethics

Pinit Ratanakul

Life and suffering

Buddhism has over 2500 years of involvement in medical theory and practice. Its health care ethics is based on its teachings concerning life, suffering, death, and compassion. The following explanation is written within the context of Thai Buddhism but shares much in common with Buddhism worldwide.

From the time of the early *sangha* or monastic communities, Buddhist monks have expressed their compassion through the practice of medicine. The Buddhist perspective on life and death cannot be truly understood apart from the Buddhist laws of causality *(paticcasamuppada)* and mutation. The relation between "cause" and "effect" in the Buddhist law of causality, also referred to as the law of conditionality, is that of the earlier to the later phase of a single process. In this context life is an interdependent process of causes and effects, arising, existing, and continuing by the concatenation of psycho-physical factors *(nama-rupa)* mutually conditioning one another. This life process has no beginning or end and is specifically referred to as the *kamma* process or the endless cycle of rebirths *(samsara).*[1] Death is considered an integral part of existence and is one phase of this cycle. In no sense is death seen as terminating the cycle.

In addition to the cause–effect nature of life, Buddhism also emphasizes its impermanence (*anicca*) and insubstantiality *(anatta)* through another law of mutation. According to this law everything, whether physical or mental, is by nature transitory and in a constant state of change. Whatever rises must fall. This state of change must thereby result in decline and decay. This is also applied to the life process in which the apparent unity of existence is divided into five aggregates (*khandhas*, the bits and pieces of muscle and bone, feelings, perceptions, impulses, and the consciousness that make up our personality), each with three traits: arising, remaining, and passing away.[2] Owing to this ephemeral nature, life is quite brief and fleeting. But no matter how brief life is, it should be lived fruitfully so that there are no regrets.

Along with the frailty and insecurity of life, it is believed that at the centre of existence there is a void. This void is the result of the insubstantial nature of life, and the aggregates, though forming a recognizable and perceivable object, do not produce a substance. All of them are insubstantial and the apparent sameness (identity) is actually the continuity of preceding causes and subsequent effects. Accordingly, for Buddhism the term "self" or Ego is a name for the linkage of all five aggregates, just as the term "human being" refers to an aggregate of body and mind. Devoid of a substantial Ego, life is like a bubble, with its centre a void.

Apart from its conditionality (cause–effect) and ephemerality, life is suffering (*dukha*). Suffering is used in Buddhism in a broader meaning to include pain, grief, misery, and dissatisfaction. All these elements of suffering are inherent in the experience of living and cannot be avoided. Owing to this reality, Buddhism concludes that human existence is insecure, fragile, and filled with suffering. The very transitory nature of life is the main cause of suffering, for even happiness is seen to be temporary. While experiencing happiness – which by definition is the absence of pain – one has expectations of the continuation of the state of joy. But these expectations can never be met. The objects of pleasure cannot last long, for they contain within themselves the potential for change and decay. Having undergone change and decay, they cease to give us happiness in their new forms. Although, like happiness, suffering is subject to change and the painful side of experience usually outweighs happiness. But despite this imbalance, life is still precious and the first precept of Buddhism prohibits the taking of life. Within this precept all killing for whatever reason is not allowed. The precept upholds the preciousness of life of all human beings regardless of the conditions of their lives. As a rule suicide is prohibited. If one destroys one's life in such a way, the great object of one's existence is lost. It is difficult to be born as a human being. In the Buddhist view only human beings can liberate themselves from *samsara*, the cycle of birth, death, and rebirth. Thus even when one is suffering from a painful and incurable disease, or when one's life is unsatisfactory, one should bear it quietly and patiently while simultaneously trying to rid oneself of the pain and suffering in all possible ways.[3]

Dying and death

As already mentioned, death is an essential part of the human predicament. It is one of the conditioned and conditioning factors of the cycle of causes and effects. Buddhism defines death in terms of the concept of impermanence and insubstantiality. Death is seen as the dissolution of the five aggregates, the psychophysical factors constituting the individual. As the manifestation of the impermanence of life, death is not a one-time event but occurs at every moment of life. Since the aggregates are in a state of constant flux, birth and death are always present in juxtaposition to each other. These momentary lives and deaths are one phase of the endless life cycle. From one perspective death is the passing away. But from another perspective death is nothing but the arising of the new state in place of the preceding one. This may be explained by means of the analogy of a door. To those who are outside the room the door is an entrance whereas to those inside the room it is an exit. But for both it is the same door. Similarly the preceding state in the cause–effect life continuum is called birth (life) whereas its following state is viewed as death, although both of them belong to the same single process. It is through an understanding of death that we can understand life. Buddhism thus sees the attempt made by people to find the meaning of life as an attempt to define the meaning of death. A man who defines death merely as an unbroken cause–effect life continuum should be able to rid himself of anxiety and then could live life to the fullest conquering the vicissitudes of life.

Buddhism agrees with the generally negative view that death is the fearful and disastrous culmination of an existence already marred by sorrow and suffering. This tragedy of death is magnified by the certainty of rebirth (again arising) and the repetition of suffering and death (passing away) in the endless life cycle. That we are locked in this cycle is an indication of the fundamental emptiness of existence. This imprisonment, however, is the result of one's own deeds (*kamma*), good or bad. It is therefore within the power of each individual to either remain in the endless cycle or to escape from it. Buddhism places death at the heart of the human predicament while also recognizing it as the primary solution to this predicament. Liberation from this human predicament is possible only by confronting death. Therefore Buddhism does not condone a melancholic reaction to the death of those dear to us. What is necessary when death occurs is that we understand its meaning and cope with it in a realistic and intelligent manner.

As a means of solving the predicament of death, Buddhism has developed special systematic techniques (meditative methods) called *moranasati* and *asubha bhavana* to enable us to face the fact of our death with equanimity and understanding and ultimately to obtain *nibbana* in which there is neither life nor death. These meditations are concentrated on the idea of death and the actual observation of the decomposing corpse. The meditator is led towards control and freedom through the revealing impermanence and insubstantial nature of existence. Freedom is obtained when one frees oneself from the clutch of the illusory Ego and its selfish desires and ultimately from the endless life cycle.[4]

As we have seen in the discussion on the concept of life, Buddhism considers every moment of life of great importance, for it is the moment in which one constructs one's own destiny. More emphasis, however, is on the last moment of life, or the dying process, in which all the five aggregates of existence are disintegrating. In Buddhist thought, in this last moment the last stage of consciousness *(cuti vinnana)* of one's life is passing away to give place to a new state *(patisondhi vinnana)*, which will form another life by its new association with the new aggregates of existence. Even if the character of the new life is affected by the whole previous life, the nature of the last conscious state still contributes significantly to the quality of the ensuing one. If it is wholesome *(kusala)*, this will produce a wholesome inauguration of the new life. Similarly, if it is unwholesome *(akusala)*, the ensuing new life will be unwholesomely inaugurated. *Consequently it is of great importance that the mind of the dying never be impaired by analgesics or sedatives.* Impairment by drugs would affect the consciousness of the dying person and make it impossible to fill his mind with wholesome thoughts.

The ideal of compassion

Compassion *(metta)* is a central moral ideal in Buddhism. It is not a sentiment or an emotion. Rather it is a universal and dispassionate love conjoined with knowledge. It radiates in the mind as a result of the recognition of human vulnerability to pain and suffering and the realization of the illusory nature of the Ego or the "I" that begets all forms of self-seeking desires. Such recognition of the human condition and the dissolution of selfhood and egoism are necessary means for the cultivation of genuine compassion that will enable us to consecrate ourselves to others. It is by these means that the mind is capable of opening itself to the needs and perspectives of others and is able to love them as they really are and respect them in their true being.

Implications for health care ethics associated with the beginning and end of life

The Buddhist view of persons in terms of psychosomatic unity and individual differences *(kamma)* implies that in the doctor–patient relationship the patient is to be treated both as a whole person and a unique individual. As such, his or her values, customary beliefs, and religious perspectives should be respected unless serious moral reasons can be given for not doing so. Similarly one's uniqueness, i.e. one's freedom of self-determination or one's ability to make oneself *(kamma)*, ought to be appreciated. This emphasis, however, does not mean that Buddhism exalts the supremacy of individual autonomy and rights, and addresses moral issues with excessively individual interpretations. The Buddhist law of conditionality links individual autonomy to social relationships based on mutuality and interdependence. In such relationships duties and obligations are more appreciated than individual rights. Although one has to make one's own life decisions, being in the world of interwoven causes and effects, one is obliged to consider the potential effects of one's decisions on other people who might suffer from them. After such consideration, the ultimate decisions are one's own. But being with the other requires one to strive for a balance of dignity, needs, duties, and responsibilities between oneself and other individuals. One will thus remake oneself by limiting one's own freedom of self-determination and will not make excessive claims on another's life and rights.[5]

Apart from conjoining the notion of individual autonomy with the concept of conditionality, Buddhism upholds the preciousness of human life irrespective of its stage of development. Even when human life manifests itself minutely, it is still precious, and destruction of it is a transgression of the first precept against killing. The whole question of whether the fetus is a person at a particular stage of development does not arise for Buddhism. A stage when personhood is or is not present cannot be distinguished because the physical and the mental are interdependent. Life is life at any given moment, no matter whether it is a simple zygote or a more complex fetus. This is the underlying reason why Buddhism is against procedures that involve the destruction of unwanted embryos.

In accordance with the great importance Buddhism assigns to the last stage of life, special care should be given to the dying to enable them to die a "good death", meaning death with a good rebirth or without rebirth (*nibbana*, enlightenment or release). In this special care, the dying should be maintained at a level of pain relief which does not impair their faculties or cloud their consciousness, but permits them to fill their minds with wholesome thoughts and/or to die before death – i.e. the disintegration of the physical and psychical aggregates that make up the personality – through inner transformation, thus enabling the dying one to let go of life without clinging and grasping. In Buddhist countries this spiritual care is reflected in rituals and symbols. In Thailand, for example, one important ritual is the reciting of a passage from the Buddhist scriptures called *Bojjhonga* with the purpose of assisting the dying to become fully conscious so as to be able to see the impermanent, unsatisfactory, and insubstantial nature of existence, as well as to fill their minds with wholesome thought. Another important ritual is the putting of a Buddha image before a dying patient and/or asking him or her to repeat the sacred word "Buddha" as a symbolic way of taking the Buddha as a refuge.

It should be noted that the Buddhist emphasis on *kamma* does not rule out the concept of justice. Although there is no equality among people because of their individual differences *(kamma),* as fellow human beings they are equals and deserve non-discriminatory, impartial treatment. Since there are morally relevant differences between people, in the context of health care justice means fairness and involves proportionate treatment. Fairness does not mean that the same amount of medical resources must be expended on all people regardless of their conditions or health needs. Rather it requires society to spend more on the poor and the disadvantaged than on other groups within society, because these people have greater need for health care services and their basic health needs have not been adequately met. Therefore there should be more medical facilities and more doctors and nurses sent to the areas – rural or urban – of greater medical need.[6]

While recognizing justice as an important moral imperative in health care, Buddhism gives compassion a central place in its ethics. After all it was compassion that originated the practice of medicine – service to suffering humanity, those afflicted in body and mind. In health care, compassion signifies two obligations that health care providers have towards their patients. One is to do all they can to enhance the health and well-being of patients and to benefit them. The second obligation is to do no further harm to those already experiencing the harm of pain and helplessness, of disease, disability, and dying. In this case compassion implies that health care providers are to seek to prevent harm (ill health and death) if it is within their power to do so; if they cannot prevent harm or pain and suffering, then they ought to seek to remove it (cure the disease, restore to health); and if they cannot remove it, their obligation is to alleviate it, lessen it (i.e. relieve the suffering, care for and comfort the dying, and maintain as best they can those beyond their capacity to cure). This practice of compassion in health care can involve self-sacrifice on the part of health care providers. It means giving time and energy and a reversal of priorities even at the cost of one's own comfort and benefit. This practice, however, has its limits in terms of meeting the needs of patients. The limits are reached when the expectations of patients are beyond the professional capacity of the health care providers or against their ethical convictions. For example, a request for open heart surgery cannot be met by a doctor who is not a heart surgeon. A doctor may also refuse to act on his patient's request, for example, to perform an abortion or assist a suicide when such a request is against his professional and/or personal ethics.

Similarly, in the case of a patient in a persistent vegetative state, health care providers may refuse to prolong the treatment indefinitely when such treatment is futile and inordinately burdensome to the patient and his or her relatives.[7] The provision of such service should be considered in terms of fairness to other patients' needs. Compassion should not be given only to a particular person but to all suffering people. In suffering and death people are equal. Compassion, in this sense, embraces justice. To render justice is a social form of compassion in recognizing others as moral equals, in giving and claiming for each other what is due as a fellow human being. In some cases compassion may mean permitting the hopelessly ill patients to die naturally, unhooked to machines, subject to no experimental treatments merely to gain scientific knowledge, not kept alive merely to be studied or to allow interns to practise on them, but following their expressed wishes to decide, as their last human act, the manner of their own dying. This "allowing to die" is believed to be different from the act of killing even if it is mercy killing. It is also different from the case where parents passively allow children to die by not giving them available food. But whether this is against the first precept is still being debated among Buddhists. The majority of them regard such cases as in a grey area where the decision between "right" and "wrong", "moral" and "immoral" is blurred. In this twilight zone mitigating factors such as the motivations behind the deed are of primary significance, the hard choices to be made between greater and lesser harms/good and the nature of the suffering of all involved. However, it is clear that Buddhism is against euthanasia – the quick, supposedly merciful ending of life to relieve pain. With regard to the argument that one is seeking to hasten the death of another in order to be merciful or to show loving kindness, Buddhism considers this a form of paternalism and self-deception. People have different pain thresholds and psychological, emotional, and spiritual factors play a great part in how much pain or suffering people can endure. People can endure pain if they find meaning in it. We might think that another is suffering unendurable pain and therefore ought to die. In this we are paternalistically imposing our values upon them. We would not want to go on living in such circumstances. But this does not mean that this painful life is meaningless to them. Besides, in Buddhist psychology, the felt desire to end another's suffering may be derived from our own inability to cope with it and our own anguish in watching another suffer. What we actually want is to save ourselves from further suffering, not them. Instead of euthanasia, Buddhist compassion leads to a different approach. What is owed to the dying is care, comfort, consolation, and companionship. Medical professionals are expected to preserve and prolong the life of all patients under their care, but when death becomes imminent, they ought to become graceful acceptors of the inevitable and turn their full attention to the compassionate care of the dying, their main concern being to relieve the suffering of patients and families and ensure a "good death".

Notes

1. The term *samsara* refers to the round of life and death in which the whole range of sentient beings, from the tiniest insect to humans, is believed to exist. Only the human being, however, has the potential to terminate this endless cycle by obtaining release or *nibbana*.

2. These five aggregates are sometimes given in a threefold scheme: (i) physical (*rupa*) : (ii) sensory perception and reaction (*vedana. sanna,* and *sankhara*) : (iii) consciousness (*vinnana*). In this case the three groups are called *rupa, cetasika* (conditioning factors of consciousness), and *citta* (state of consciousness). The five aggregates are also arranged in two groups: (i) *rupa* (ii) *nama* (the other four aggregates). For more details, see Edward Conze, 1970, *Buddhist Thought in India,* Ann Arbor: University of Michigan Press, 107ff.

3. Yet in some cases, according to Buddhist Scriptures, taking one's own life is sometimes allowed for noble ends. The giving of one's own life to save the lives of the others as a Bodhisatta (a Buddha-to-be) gave himself to a hungry lioness to save her from eating her own clubs is one example of this exception. This event in the Jatakas Stories, the collection of the stories of the Buddha's previous lives, is usually used by some Buddhists to justify suicide, for example, in the case of Thic Quang-Due, a Vietnamese monk, who burned himself to death to oppose the Diem regime in 1963. In one Buddhist text *(Samuvutta-Nikaya)* the Buddha was said to give approval to the suicide of a monk named Godhika who, after attaining the state of spiritual release through meditation six times in succession and then, because of incurable illness, falling away from it, committed suicide the seventh time he attained it, in order not to fall away from it again.

4. The teaching of *nibbana* as the practically attainable goal of man's struggle to escape from life, suffering, and death prevents Buddhism from being a "religion of despair". There are various meanings of *nibbana* found in different contexts in Buddhist texts. In this discussion the term is used to mean the unconditioned state of consciousness in which there is the ceasing of the "I" (Ego), lust, hatred, and delusion, the three principal forms of evil in Buddhism. This state is not caused, not originated. It simply makes itself known when all that is opposite (ego-absorption, lust, hatred, and delusion) is removed. There are two kinds of *nibbana* : *sa-upatisesa nibbana-nibbana* with the total extinction of greed (*lobha*), hatred (*dosa*), and delusion (*moha*) but without the disintegration of all the five aggregates of

existence, and *anu-patisesanibbana-nibbana* without any element of life remaining. It is believed that with this state of consciousness completely void of any defilement a person lives not for himself, but for others and with death is released from the round of existence. This liberating wisdom (*vijja*) is thus like the indispensable key that unlocks the chains binding us to the wheel of life, death, and rebirth.

5. For a Buddhist critique of the Western concept of autonomy see Pinit Ratanakul, 1994, "Community and Compassion: A Theravada Buddhist look at principlism" in *A matter of principles: Ferment in U.S. bioethics,* ed. Edwin R. Dubose et al. Valley Forge: Trinity Press International.

6. This concept of justice and other Buddhist health care ethical principles are discussed in Pinit Ratanakul "Bioethics in Thailand: The struggle for Buddhist solutions", *The Journal of Medicine and Philosophy* 13, 1988.

7. For more discussion on the issue, see Keown Damien, 1995, *Buddhism and bioethics.* London: St. Martin Press.

Chapter 8
Chinese Health Care Ethics

Edwin Hui

Chinese worldview and presuppositions

In all schools of traditional Chinese philosophy, the universe is regarded as a unity which consists of three interacting and interdependent members: heaven, earth, and man.[1] The ultimate basis of this unity of nature is provided by the *Dao* which as the first indeterminate principle is the primal origin from which all things become determinate.[2,3,4] *Dao* runs through everything in the universe and directs a self-evolving process through which multiplicity is derived from unity.[5,6] *Dao* is not considered to be a god or deity and is without a will, and it is through its intrinsic creative force that all created beings and things are generated naturally and spontaneously. Because nature is united in the *Dao*, and human life ultimately comes from and returns to nature, the Chinese believe that one's life is connected to or united with nature; and this has formally become a doctrine called *t'ien jen ho yi* (Heaven and Human are One) which requires among other things that man's life and conduct in life should conform to the rhythms of nature.

Concretely, in the universe *Dao* is expressed through the operations of "*ch'i*", "*yin–yang*" and "*wu-hsing*" (five phases).[7] The concept of *ch'i*[8] conveys the idea of a life-giving material force which pervades heaven and earth and is dispersed to the other members of the created world for growth and sustenance.[9,10] Chuang Tze (399-295 BCE) said, "A human life is formed because the material force (*ch'i*) is being gathered up; when [*ch'i* is being] gathered, life results; when dispersed, death ensues."[11] When one dies, the material force (*ch'i*) that is being dispersed is reunited with the material force (*ch'i*) of the cosmos from which it originally came. In human conception, it is believed that during fetal development, the *ch'i* is further distributed to the different visceral organs of the body so that the cosmos, the person, and the body organs can be seen as connected through the media of *ch'i* to become a holistic entity.[12] Furthermore, the *ch'i* exists with a certain rhythm and volatility and is regulated by two principles, "*yin*" and "*yang*".[13,14] This cyclical movements of *yin* and *yang* is reinforced by the theory of *wu-hsing* or Five Phases elements which provides the important concept of rotation and succession[15] so that together they co-operate to bring about the perpetual cycles of the various phenomena of the world, e.g. birth–death–rebirth, spring–winter–spring and so on. Combining the "two" with the "five" serves to emphasize the dynamic and orderly nature of the law of operation of the universe, so that in the final analysis, one may say that the material force (*ch'i*), operating according to the rhythms of *yin-yang* and the "*wu-hsing*", expresses and actualizes the operation of the *Dao*.

The Chinese conception of human personhood

The person as a psychosomatic unity

Traditional Chinese philosophy recognizes that human life is made up of two essential components: "*hsing*" (body, form) and "*shen*" (psyche, spirit); both are derived from the material force *ch'i* and are related to each other. When the two elements (psyche and body) are in harmony, the person lives; but if they are in disharmony, the person will not live.[16] Subsequent development of the whole system of traditional Chinese medicine has been based on the interactions and functions of the physical and psychical elements in the human person. For example, it is believed that the secret to avoiding disease and illness is to ensure the unimpeded circulation of the "psychic energy" in the body. It is also believed that different "psychic energies" in the various organs of the body must be preserved if health is to be maintained (Huang Ti, 23). The notion that one's essential psychical forces are found inside bodily organs explains partly why Chinese people are generally resistant to surgical intervention, for they fear that if the abdomen is surgically opened, the various forces or energies will escape out of the body.[17] It also explains why Chinese people are generally reluctant to donate organs for transplant, for they fear that the psychological or spiritual elements which reside in the organs may be given away when they may have post-mortem significance. Maintaining the "psychic energies" is of paramount importance because ultimately it is these psychical forces which contribute to human consciousness, will, purpose, and the sense of justice that distinguish humans from animals. Here we observe an apparent convergence of the minds of the East and West in the emphasis of a person's consciousness and rationality which has assumed great importance in the definition of personhood in modern Western thought.

The person as a social and moral agent

In contrast to the more individualistic definition of human personhood heavily influenced by Daoism, the dominant Confucian philosophy insistently defines human personhood in social and moral terms. In the Confucian tradition, a person is never seen as an isolated individual but is always conceived of as a centre of relationships;[18] a person is always a "person-in-relations".[19] The bulk of the Confucian ethical teaching of self-cultivation of an individual person is carried out in a social context and for the purpose of fulfilling social responsibility. A person's nature is actualized only through human relatedness. It may be said that relation has ontological significance in Confucian anthropology. It both constitutes and completes personhood.

The principle of *jen*, family, and social hierarchy

In the Chinese Confucian tradition, human relations are regulated by the principle of *jen*, which has been variously translated as benevolence, humanity, humanness, and compassion. But fundamentally *jen* is a relational term and is used to describe the relational or social nature of persons. Negatively put, the principle of *jen* requires that you "Do not do to others what you do not want them to do to you".[20] In positive terms, it states that "A man of humanity (*jen*), wishing to establish his own character, also establishes the character of others, and wishing to be prominent himself, also helps others to be prominent".[21] As such *jen* includes all virtues and a person is only a person when he fulfils the principle of *jen*.[22] In the actual implementation of the principle of *jen* in human relations in Chinese society, Confucians have adopted a rigidly hierarchical structure, known as the "Five Relations", which encompasses all interactions in society: that between (i) father and son, (ii) ruler and minister, (iii) old (superior) and young (inferior), (iv) husband and wife, and (v) friends. A rigid set of rules of propriety, affection, righteousness, faithfulness, etc, collectively known as *li* are elaborated to regulate these relations.[23] All conduct in Chinese society is essentially governed by this set of rules which, if fully complied with, fulfils the principle of *jen*. In particular these rules are applied in order to maintain the family as the most fundamental unit in social organization. For example, the Rules of Propriety (*li*) mandate that the predominant affections for parents are kindness and rightness; for children towards parents, "*hsiao*" (filial piety) is the appropriate attitude; and for younger siblings towards their older siblings, "*ti*" (brotherly respect) is the proper disposition. In sum what Confucianism wants to emphasize is that when everybody accepts one's role and discharges one's duty in accordance with that "named" role in the various family relationships, then family order will be secured. Once the roles are differentiated, hierarchically arranged, and obediently kept in the family, then a similar hierarchy can be justified in a wider social context to promote social solidarity and harmony. From the viewpoint of health care ethics, it may be of interest to note that the Confucian teaching of filial piety is explicitly expressed in terms of the physical well-being of the parents. Children from a Confucian family are supposed to be very concerned about their parents' health,[24] and should always be attendant on their parents' physical well-being.[25]

Implications for health care decision making

Informed consent issues

The Confucian concept of social personhood, regulated by the principles of *jen* and filial piety, and organized in a social hierarchy, provides distinctive perspectives when the issue of informed consent in health care ethics is being considered. We will consider its impact from a) the patient's and b) the physician's perspectives:

a) From the patient's point of view, the notion of respect for an individual's right to self-determination is a weak notion in Chinese culture. In fact, the Confucian concept of social personhood challenges the assumption that the patient is the one to be told of the diagnosis and prognosis and to make medical decisions. When a Chinese becomes sick, her behaviour and expectation are closely tied with a strong sense of personal identification with and mutual dependence on her family. For example, it is not shameful for a Chinese elderly sick person to be dependent on her children, but rather it is something to which she is entitled. According to the *Book of Rites*, the rules are: "When a ruler is ill, and has to drink medicine, the minister first tastes it. The same is the rule for a son and an ailing parent."[26] In the Confucian social hierarchy, the elderly sick person can expect to be cared for by her family, and her sick role includes the privilege to be relieved of a large share of personal responsibility, including most of the decision making process of her own medical care, even though the patient may be rational and competent. Family members, especially the patient's children, are expected to take over that responsibility and assume the various roles of being children, caregiver, protector, and surrogate decision maker. In other words, whereas family input is usually not determinative in the West, in the Chinese culture family input is often decisive; a one-to-one patient–physician encounter is rare and family members are expected to be invited in at all times, making the conventional requirement of patient informed consent not easily enforceable. Even psychiatrists report that one expects parents to come with adult patients. Specifically patients are not to be told the news of a terminal illness because from a Confucian point of view, governed by the rule of filial piety, it is considered morally inexcusable to disclose terminal illness which may add further harm to the patient. To fulfil filial piety, dying elderly patients must be protected from fateful news. This is at odds with the Western notion of full disclosure of relevant information to the patient.

b) From the physician's point of view, both his[27] role and function are impacted by these Confucian concepts. To start with, Confucians believe that the principle of *jen* should be the regulatory principle for the physician's character as well as his conduct just as it is for other members of the community. For this reason, a Chinese physician will likely follow the inclinations of the family to satisfy all the other social protocols inspired by the principle of *jen*, particularly the requirements of filial piety as perceived by the patient's family. On the other hand, with the hierarchical structure of a Confucian society, the physician is in a social position to override the decision of the family if he feels the need to do so. Even though the exact position of a physician is not specified in the Confucian scheme of "five relations", traditionally physicians command a respect equivalent to that of parents in the family or elders in a clan. There is a common saying in Chinese: "physicians have the heart of parents", indicating that people expect physicians to act lovingly as parents do, and accord them a level of respect commensurate with elders and parents. With this venerable status, it is not uncommon for Chinese physicians to have a paternalistic attitude in their dealings with patients. They will not find it ethically troubling to withhold information from patients if in their judgment it is not beneficial for them. As well, in keeping with the Confucian tradition, patients and their family find it quite natural to submit to the opinion of their physician. In this regard, the inclinations of a patient's family and physician act in consonance to disrespect patients' autonomy.

Beginning-of-life issues

In the Chinese conception of social personhood, the definition of a person as a "being in family relations" has significant ethical implications for beginning-of-life issues. For example, one of the most important ways to show filial piety is to provide male offspring to propagate the family name. Mencius specifically stated that, "There are three things which are unfilial, and to have no posterity is the greatest of them all."[28] This explains why births in general and male births in particular are welcome events in Chinese society. Therefore, the traditional Chinese attitude towards abortion is generally negative, especially for male fetuses if the sex of the fetus is known; and this has also been reinforced by the traditional teaching of the unity of nature in which, as we have seen, humanity is not only a member of the Heaven–Earth–Man triad, but also a product of Heaven and Earth. Life is always viewed as precious, and to take life is something to be undertaken with the utmost caution. This high view of life is supplemented with the Buddhist teaching of compassion[29] which was imported to China from India around the second century CE. Nevertheless, even with this high view of the preciousness of life, the abortion and abandonment of girls has been more common over the centuries and especially under the limits to childbirth policy in the present day PRC.

As the value of male progeny assumes a particularly important place in Chinese culture, one may expect a Chinese infertile couple to seek help from modern assisted reproductive technologies to ensure male progeny as long as the sperm comes from the husband. The use of donor eggs and the employment of surrogate mothers would probably be less desirable, but they are not of primary importance. This tradition of producing a male offspring as fulfilment of filial piety may become a strong justificatory reason to perform prenatal sex selection in contemporary China where for reasons of population control the policy of "one child per family" is being practised currently.

In contrast, the doctrine of "Heaven and Human are One" gives rise to the idea of *t'ien ming*, which literally means "heaven's destiny", i.e. life is destined by nature. On this basis, Daoism adopts a more passive attitude towards life. One of the founders of Daoism, Chuang Tze said, "Life and death are due to fate (*ming*, destiny) and their constant succession like day and night is due to Nature, beyond the interference of man."[30] This means that human actions pertaining to issues of life and death must be guided by the principle of "*wu-wei*" which literally means non-action. By "non-action", what Lao Tze (6th century? BCE) and Chuang Tze meant was not so much the absence of action, but acting without artificiality and without over-action. In this context, this teaching would probably oppose most forms of assisted reproductive technologies.

Death and dying issues

Confucius (551–479 BCE) himself accepted death as an objective fact of the end of life. He was known to have made terse, factual, and matter-of-fact pronouncements about his students' and friends' death without much explanation as if there was nothing to be explained. According to him death is regrettable and unavoidable, but death is not the most significant event in life. As *jen* (humanity, benevolence) is the most important principle guiding life, so it also regulates the significance of death. If *jen* is achieved, human personhood is fulfilled and death pales in significance.[31] "The Master said, 'He who has heard about *dao* in the morning may readily die in the evening.'"[32] Here *dao* refers to *jen*. For a Confucian, therefore, death is evaluated in terms of accomplishment in this world, i.e. the fulfilment of *jen*. A death is a "good" one, worthy and acceptable, only when most if not all of one's moral duties of life have been properly fulfilled. Any resistance to acknowledging a certain terminal illness or to foregoing futile medical treatments may mean some unfinished business perceived by the patient, and hence an effort to extend life to the last breath in order to complete one's unfinished task(s) in life.

Furthermore, the requirement of filial piety also makes a difference in the ability to acknowledge the terminal nature of an illness. For example, an elderly dying Chinese person may well be resigned to a "good death", but her children may be reluctant to grant her this wish for "good death" for reasons related to filial piety. Since filial piety can only be expressed when a parent is alive, to extend an ailing parent's life is to extend the opportunity to show filial piety. This alone is a common reason for children to reject a physician's judgment that any further medical intervention is futile and to insist that every heroic measure be taken for their dying parent. To forfeit this duty produces a strong sense of guilt and shame which is a significant reason for family members to request unreasonable life-extending measures. In addition, deeply ingrained in the Chinese mindset is a strong embodied understanding of filial piety which is expressed in the saying, "The body, including our hair and skin, we receive from our parents. We dare not cause any injury to it, and this is the beginning of filial piety".[33] That is a decisive reason why one should take care of one's health in all circumstances. This provides the notion that physical harm to one's body amounts to a violation of filial piety and accounts for many instances of persistence in medical treatment even when such treatment has been determined to be of no further medical benefit.

A Chinese person's attitude towards a dying patient is also influenced by the doctrine of "Heaven and Human are One". In the Confucian school, which has the most "this-worldly" orientation and positive attitude towards life among all the schools of Chinese philosophy, this doctrine is interpreted as man's responsibility to fulfil the full measure of life span that nature intends each one to have. "Comply to the years given by nature, one's life can be considered complete and fulfilled."[34] To give up medical treatment as futile, or to foreclose on life by euthanasia or physician-assisted suicide would incur reprimand or punishment by nature. For this reason it is a common belief among Chinese people that "It is more preferable to hang on to life, even a 'bad life', than to give oneself up to a good death". This does not mean that the Chinese have no regard for dignity in life and death; rather, "to give oneself up to a good death" is interpreted as an escape from the life span prescribed by nature. So, even when life is unbearable with much suffering, one is motivated to endure it if it means compliance to the life span predetermined by nature. Quite obviously this tradition will have significant bearings on a patient's decision whether or not to accept a particular medical intervention as futile. All in all, the Confucian interpretation of the doctrine of "Heaven and Human are One" is predominant in Chinese culture and provides a general orientation in the Chinese mindset to love life and hate death, so that until recently practices of any form of euthanasia would not have been deemed acceptable.

Drawing from Lao Tze's authoritative writings in *Tao-te-Ching*, though often taken out of context, religious Daoism suggests that the perfect man of *Dao* is immune from harm and hence potentially immortal. Lao Tze said, "He who does not lose his place (with *Dao*) will endure. He who dies but does not really perish enjoys long life."[35] From this, the beliefs of the post-mortem survival of the whole bodily person and an afterlife of torture and suffering in the Hades (Yellow Spring) were developed. To avoid these and other potential post-mortem calamities, second century religious Daoism was responsible for the first systematic experimentation in therapeutics with alchemy, diet, breathing exercises, as well as certain beneficial forms of sexual intercourse – all in the hope of maintaining youth and attaining longevity and immortality. Such was the case that by the time of the Han Dynasty (206 BCE – 220 CE) the idea of and the quest for physical immortality struck deep roots in popular thought. Thus there exists in religious Daoism a powerful tradition of Chinese thought which looks at death as an obstacle to be overcome. As a result, patients with a strong Daoist religious background may actually be fearful of their imminent death and desperately cling onto any means to extend life. In this view, any suffering associated with heroic measures of modern medicine is less intimidating than the "mountain of sharp knives and boiling oil bath"[36] believed to be awaiting them in their post-mortem existence.

As a philosophy, Daoism has a radically different teaching regarding death. It draws on the thoughts of the founder Lao Tze, who taught that a person's death, like a fallen leaf returning to its roots, is a natural phenomenon and part of a natural cycle – nothing to be afraid of. "Man comes into life and goes out to death."[37] For Chuang Tze, who made the most distinctive contribution to the Chinese understanding of death, life and death are only human distinctions made by those who do not understand the unity of all things that resides in the *Dao*.

> Life is the comrade of death, death is the beginning of life. Who understands their order? Man's life is a gathering up of material force. If it comes together, there is life; if it scatters, there is death. And if life and death are comrades to each other, then why is there suffering?"[38]

For this reason, one should think equally well of both life and death which are but two of the "ten thousand changes" of the human form over which man has no control, no ability to change, and no way to escape. Chuang Tze's thought on death is most fully revealed in a passage entitled "The Equality of Life and Death" which describes how he reacted to the death of his wife:

> Chuang Tze's wife died and Hui Tze went to offer his condolence. He found Chuang Tze squatting on the ground and singing, beating on an earthen bowl. He said, "Someone has lived with you, raised children for you and now she has aged and died. Is it not enough that you should not shed any tear? But now you sing and beat the bowl. Is this not too much?"
> "No," replied Chuang Tze. "When she died, how could I help being affected? But as I think the matter over, I realize that originally she had no life; and not only no life, she had no form; not only no form, she had no material force (*ch'i*). In the limbo of existence and non-existence, there was transformation and the material force was evolved. The material force was transformed to be form, form was transformed to become life, and now birth has transformed to become death. This is like the rotation of the four seasons, spring, summer, fall, and winter. Now she lies asleep in the great house (the universe). For me to go about weeping and wailing would be to show my ignorance of destiny. Therefore, I desist."[39]

So, for Chuang Tze, in the face of death, acceptance is the only appropriate response. Hence a patient who subscribes to philosophic Daoism is more likely to accept a medical condition pronounced as irreversible and not to demand unnecessary treatments. For such a person, life is leaving home, and death is homecoming; as a "companion of nature", dying is returning to nature and should be done in peace and with contentment. Chuang Tze says, "When we come, it is because it was the occasion to be born. When we go, it is to follow the natural course of things ... For the universe gave me the body so I may be carried, my life so I may toil, my old age so I may repose, and my death so I may rest. Therefore to regard life as good is the way to regard death as good."[40]

Notes

1. Lao Tze, 1963, Ch. 25, 56, 58, p.82; Ch. 20, 50a, p.79; Cf. Wing-tsit Chan, 1963, 153.
2. Chuang Tze, Chan 1963, 194.
3. Lao Tze, Chan, 139.
4. Ibid., 141.
5. Chuang Tze, Chuang Tze, tran. Legge, Vol. 1, p.342, quoted in Joseph Needham, 1956, 47. Also, ibid., 157.
6. Lao Tze, Chan,160.
7. These concepts are developed either simultaneously or more likely subsequent to the exposition of the concept of Dao by Lao Tze.
8. Ch'i is variously translated as material force, life force, vital force, vital energy, etc. I agree with W. T. Chan and adopt material force as the most accurate translation.
9. Chuang Tze, Chan, 209.
10. Also see Loewe, 69.
11. Chuang Tze, Ch. 22, my translation.
12. Also see "The Concept of Ch'i" in chapter 3 above.
13. The yin–yang principle is a dialectical concept which attempts to explain the various phenomena of the universe which appear to be both interdependent on and in opposition to each other: dark and light, cold and heat, rest and activity, life and death, etc. See note 6.
14. Also see "The Concept of Yin-Yang" in chapter 3 above.
15. Also see "The Theory of the Five Elements" in chapter 3 above.
16. Kuan Chung, *Kuan Tze*, Bk. XVI, Sec. 49, my translation.
17. Another important reason for a Chinese to resist surgery is the association of the fear of blood loss with the loss of an irreplaceable primordial vital force "yuan ch'i" which one inherits from one's parents.
18. Confucius, BK IX, p.83; Mencius, Bk VIA:7, p.231.
19. Mencius, 1984, IVB:19, 165. And Shun being the legendary ancient model sage-king.
20. Confucius, The Analects, 15:23, Chan, 44.
21. Confucius, The Analects, 6:28, Chan, 31.
22. Confucius, The Analects, 12:1, Chan, 38.
23. Mencius, 3A:4, Chan, 69f.
24. Confucius, The Analects, 2:6, Chan, 23.
25. Confucius, The Analects, 6:19, Chan, 33.
26. The Li Ki, Bk 1, Part III, sec. 2, Vol. XXVII, F. Max Müller 1966, 114.
27. Until modern times, all traditional physicians were male.
28. Mencius, Mencius, 4A:26, Source Book, tran. Chan, p.75.
29. See "Buddhist Health Care Ethics" by Pint Ratanakul in this volume.
30. Chuang Tze, Ch. 6, Chan, 193.
31. Confucius, Analects, 15:8, Chan, 43.
32. Ibid., 4:8, my translation.
33. *The Book on Filial Piety*, my translation.
34. Han Fei Tze, *Han Fei Tze*, my translation.
35. Lao Tze, Tao Te Ching, Ch. 33, Chan, 156.
36. Common Chinese folk saying of uncertain origin.
37. Ibid., 163.
38. Chuang Tze, Chuang Tze, Ch. 22, my translation.
39. Chuang Tze, Chuang Tze, Ch. 18, Chan, 209.
40. Ibid., 197.

References

Chan, W. T. 1963. *A source book in Chinese philosophy.* Princeton, NJ: Princeton University Press.

Confucius. 1992. *The analects.* 2nd ed. D. C. Lau, (tran.), Hong Kong, Shatin: The Chinese University Press.

Fairbank, J. K. 1957. *Chinese thought and institutions.* Chicago: The University of Chicago Press.

Huang Ti. 1970. *Nei ching su we,* (The Yellow Emperor's classic of internal medicine). Ilza Veith (tran.), Berkeley: University of California Press.

Lao Tze. 1963. *Tao te ching.* D. C. Lau (tran.) London: Penguin Books.

Loewe, M. 1994. *Chinese ideas of life and death.* Taipei: SMC Publishing Inc.

Mencius. 1984. *Mencius.* D. C. Lau, (tran.) Hong Kong, Shatin: The Chinese University Press.

Müller, F. M. (ed.). 1966. "The Li Ki", James Legge (tran.) *in The sacred book of the East,* Vol. XXVII, Delhi: Motilal Banarsidass.

Needham, J. 1956. *Science and civilisation in China.* Vol. 2, Cambridge: Cambridge University Press.

Northrop, F.S.C. (ed.). 1949. *Ideological differences and world order.* New Haven: Yale University Press.

Chapter 9
Secular Health Care Ethics

Barry Hoffmaster

The early, formative contributions to contemporary health care ethics in North America came principally from theologians. Reflecting on "the birth of bioethics", Robert Veatch observes:

> It is striking how many of the scholars and leaders in those early years were trained in theology, especially Protestant theology ... Important themes of rights and the affirmation of the lay decisionmaker read directly, I would suggest, from Protestant theological themes. (Veatch 1993, S7)

The movement was, however, quickly secularized. Daniel Callahan, a co-founder of The Hastings Center over twenty-five years ago, believes that the acceptance of health care ethics in America was gained only by jettisoning its religious heritage: "... the first thing that those in bioethics had to do – though I don't believe anyone set this as a conscious agenda – was to push religion aside" (Callahan 1993, S8).

Law and philosophy replaced theology. Law provided a rich source of seminal cases, about matters such as refusal of treatment, the termination of life, and surrogate motherhood, that have in large part defined contemporary health care ethics but at the same time have emphasized its overwhelmingly reactive nature. Ethics, as Arthur Caplan points out, is constantly "struggling to keep up with technology. No matter how hard you think and no matter what you do, you're trailing behind Dr Edwards, Dr Jarvik, Dr Bailey, or Dr Starzl" (Caplan 1993, S15). While law provided much content for secular health care ethics, philosophy, in its Anglo-American analytic mode, gave it structure:

> ... twenty-five to thirty years ago, medical ethics was hardly even individuated as a field. It was a mixture of religion, whimsy, exhortation, legal precedents, various traditions, philosophies of life, miscellaneous moral rules, and epithets (uttered by either wise or witty physicians) ... [P]hilosophy provided the push toward systematization, consistency, and clarity, as progress within medicine increasingly erupted into moral dilemmas. The maneuvers, ploys, and strategies of philosophy have been important for bringing system and organization to medical ethics. It asks probing and organizing questions; it understands how to discover and work with assumptions, implications, and foundations. (Clouser 1993, S10)

What gave contemporary health care ethics a point, however, was the goal of affirming patients' rights, in particular, the right to decide about their own health care. Veatch sees this theme embedded in the theological origins of health care ethics, but its congruence with liberal political ideology is one of the factors to which Callahan attributes the success of health care ethics:

> The final factor of great importance [to the acceptance of bioethics] ... was the emergence ideologically of a form of bioethics that dovetailed very nicely with the reigning political liberalism of the educated classes in America. Politically America has always been a liberal society, as manifested by the market system economically and by a great emphasis on individual freedom in our cultural and political institutions. Bioethics came along with the kind of intellectual agenda that was wholly compatible with that of liberalism. (Callahan 1993, S8)

The hallmark of that liberalism in health care ethics is the freedom of individual patients to make voluntary, informed decisions about the care they receive.

Traditionally physicians, by virtue of their training and clinical experience, have been regarded as knowing what is best for their patients and thus entitled to make decisions on their behalf. But contemporary health care ethics has at least in theory wrested that authority from physicians and vested it in patients. The legal manifestation of this shift is the emergence of the doctrine of informed consent. The philosophical manifestation is the rejection of physician paternalism and the establishment of patient autonomy or patient self-determination (Buchanan 1978). Two considerations have been influential in bringing about this shift. One is the recognition that clinical decisions are as much about values as they are about matters of fact. Even if physicians are "experts" with respect to the facts, they are not with respect to their patients' values, and thinking that they are commits what has been called the "fallacy of the generalization of expertise" (Veatch 1973). Because patients know their own values best, they are in the best position to determine what decisions accord with their values. The other is the appreciation that it is patients, not doctors, who live with the consequences of clinical decisions. Whatever decision is made affects the patient most directly, most intimately, and most profoundly. For that reason as well decision making should be the responsibility of the patient.

This issue of who should decide was and continues to be framed in terms of various models of the physician–patient relationship. In 1972 Robert Veatch distinguished the engineering model, the priestly model, the collegial model, and the contractual model, and argued in favour of the contractual model of physician and patient roles, in part because "in this contractual context patient control of decision-making in the individual level is assured without the necessity of insisting that the patient participate in every trivial decision" (Veatch 1972, 7). In 1992 Ezekiel Emanuel and Linda Emanuel described four models of the physician–patient relationship: the paternalistic model, the informative model, the interpretative model, and the deliberative model (Emanuel and Emanuel 1992). They recognize that different models will be appropriate in different clinical situations, but they opt for the deliberative model as the ideal for the physician–patient relationship. Their preference for the deliberative model relies in part on how they understand the notion of patient autonomy:

> Freedom and control over medical decisions alone do not constitute patient autonomy. Autonomy requires that individuals critically assess their own values and preferences; determine whether they are desirable; affirm, upon reflection, these values as ones that should justify their actions; and then be free to initiate action to realize the values. The process of deliberation integral to the deliberative model is essential for realizing patient autonomy understood in this way. (Emanuel and Emanuel 1992, 2225)

The deliberative model takes seriously the notion that physicians are supposed to be teachers. Physicians should engage their patients in discussions about what values are important to them and get them to appraise those values and determine how they impinge upon the medical decisions confronting them. Physicians do not simply defer to the requests or decisions patients make, as a simple-minded notion of patient autonomy could suggest. Rather, they collaborate with their patients and prompt them to reflect on what decisions are best for them. This more active role could, as

Emanuel and Emanuel recognize, slide into paternalism:

> ... no doubt, in practice, the deliberative physician may occasionally lapse
> into paternalism. However, like the ideal teacher, the deliberative physician
> attempts to *persuade* the patient of the worthiness of certain values, not to
> *impose* those values paternalistically; the physician's aim is not to subject the
> patient to his or her will, but to persuade the patient of a course of action as
> desirable. (Emanuel and Emanuel 1992, 2225)

Although differences exist about exactly what patient autonomy means, and
thus about what respecting patient autonomy requires in specific situations,
the dominant position in contemporary health care ethics abjures paternalism
and protects the authority of patients to make decisions about their own care.

This position, of course, assumes that patients are competent. But the
notion of autonomy also guides decision making on behalf of incompetent
patients. The prevailing view in health care ethics is that a proxy decision
maker, the person authorized to decide on behalf of someone who is not
competent, should adopt the "substituted judgment" approach, that is, should
try to decide as the incompetent person would were he or she capable of
doing so. Only if that is impossible, because the incompetent person was
never able to form or never expressed relevant views, should the proxy
decision maker decide on the basis of what is in that person's best interest.
The development of living wills or advance directives, which set out the
wishes of competent persons about the kinds of medical treatment they
would and would not want if they were in a variety of circumstances and no
longer competent to make decisions themselves, is yet another manifestation
of respect for patient autonomy.

Probably the most noteworthy and distinctive feature of contemporary
health care ethics is this widespread endorsement of patient autonomy. The
moral issue of whether physicians or patients should have the authority to
make health care decisions has been settled in favour of the individualistic
values that characterize what Callahan calls the ideology of political
liberalism. Vesting decision making authority in patients is indeed a valuable
contribution of contemporary health care ethics. This emphasis on individual
freedom and the right to make decisions has, however, had the unfortunate
consequence of unduly restricting the focus of much of health care ethics.
And now the problems resulting from an ethos of patient autonomy are
emerging.

One thorny issue concerns the limits of patient autonomy. On what
grounds may health care professionals legitimately say "no" to patient
requests or demands? If a patient demands an antibiotic for what the doctor
confidently believes is a viral infection, or if a relative demands that life
support be continued when the health care team feels that further aggressive

interventions are "futile" and perhaps even harmful to the patient, how may these apparently autonomous requests be refused? May health care professionals say "no" because, for example, their personal or professional integrity would be violated, because the treatment would be expensive, or because they feel the treatment would not be in the best interest of the patient? Respect for autonomy is an important value in health care, but it is not the only value, and it is not always the most important value.

Another difficult issue concerns the extent to which the interests of a patient's family should be considered (Blustein 1993; Hardwig 1990). One argument for respecting patient autonomy, as we have seen, is that it is the patient who is most profoundly affected by whatever decision is made. But in many cultures, the identity of the patient may be understood in collective or "we-self" terms. Even patients who think of themselves as individuals often do not live in isolation. Their families are also affected, sometimes in momentous ways, by decisions about their care, particularly as more and more health care is being shifted out of hospitals and institutions and into homes and communities. The burden of providing that care then falls upon members of a patient's family, generally wives, mothers, and daughters. But why does the same argument that is invoked to give patients the authority to make decisions about their care not also apply to family members who are affected by that care? By parity of reasoning, if a decision is likely to have a profound impact on the life of a relative, should that relative not have a say in the decision?

Figuring out how to do that is of course not easy. How much say should a relative have? Could a relative who felt that the burden of care would be too onerous override or veto a patient's decision? How should relatives in "we-self" cultures participate in the decision making process? Should their participation be restricted to a family conference with the health care team, or should they be allowed a more extensive role? And what about the effect on the patient? Would a patient who is ill and vulnerable to begin with, and who depends on family members for care, be in any position to disagree with what family members want? The practical problems in extending decision making authority to families are challenging. The general point that emerges from this matter, however, is that health care decision making must be put in a broader context. Focusing simply on the physician–patient dyad leaves out much that is morally relevant. In a hospital it is not simply the doctor but also other members of the health care team who are involved in and affected by decisions. And at home it is not simply the patient but also members of the patient's family who live with the consequences of decisions and may participate in the patient's self-identity. The scope of health care ethics needs to expand beyond physician and patient and encompass the circumstances and settings in which decisions arise and are made.

Once that is done, however, features of the institutional, social, cultural, and political contexts within which decision making occurs become decidedly relevant to health care ethics. With respect to institutional factors, for example, Renee Anspach has shown how the ways in which the jobs of physicians and nurses are structured in a neonatal intensive care unit can influence the different perceptions those physicians and nurses have of the prognoses for seriously ill new-borns and consequently their views about whether aggressive treatment of those new-borns is warranted (Anspach 1993). Economic considerations, such as what treatments are funded by a provincial health insurance plan in Canada or what drugs are included in the formulary approved by a health maintenance organization in the United States, impose constraints on the range of what can be decided. Economic considerations also have an enormous impact on access to health care when care is largely provided by the private sector, as it is in the United States.

Questions about power likewise arise in this broader perspective. Feminist approaches to health care ethics are particularly concerned with questions of male domination and female subordination, as exemplified for example by the struggles of women to cope with artificial reproductive technologies or of nurses to escape the traditional hegemony of physicians. Discrimination against women is particularly hard to rectify and eliminate, however, because, as Susan Sherwin argues, it "is embedded in the fabric of our culture" and the ways in which the interests of women are "systematically subordinated" are "so extensive, so familiar, and so entrenched in our habits of thought that it is possible not to notice them at all" (Sherwin 1992, 13). A feminist approach to health care ethics consequently is less concerned with moral decisions and moral quandaries and more concerned with exposing the ways in which a health care system and the social arrangements within which it operates perpetuate the exploitation and oppression of women. Identifying and transforming the power structures that oppress women in the health care system requires a more sweeping and penetrating moral analysis than results from an examination of physician–patient interactions.

A similarly expansive analysis is required to identify and assess the role of cultural factors in health care ethics. Such an approach can build on, but needs to proceed well beyond, what has been accomplished in contemporary health care ethics so far. Some of the issues that need to be addressed in that fuller analysis are outlined in the concluding section of Part II, as a transition to the discussions of specific problems and policies that follow.

References

Anspach, R. R. 1993. *Deciding who lives*. Berkeley: University of California Press.
Blustein, J. 1993. The family in medical decisionmaking. *Hastings Center Report* 23, 3, 6-

13.

Buchanan, A. 1978. Medical paternalism. *Philosophy and Public Affairs* 7, 370-390.

Callahan, D. 1993. Why America accepted bioethics. *Hastings Center Report* 23, 6 (Suppl.), S8-S9.

Caplan, A. L. 1993. What bioethics brought to the public. *Hastings Center Report* 23, 6 (Suppl.), S14-S15.

Clouser, K. D. 1993. Bioethics and philosophy. *Hastings Center Report* 23, 6 (Suppl.), S10-S11.

Emanuel, E. J. & Emanuel, L. L. 1992. Four models of the physician–patient relationship. *JAMA* 267, 2221-2226.

Hardwig, J. 1990. What about the family? *Hastings Center Report* 20, 2, 5-10.

Sherwin, S. 1992. *No Longer Patient.* Philadelphia: Temple University Press.

Veatch, R. M. 1972. Models for ethical medicine in a revolutionary age. *Hastings Center Report* 2,3, 5-7.

Veatch, R. M. 1973. Generalization of expertise. *Hastings Center Studies, 1,2,* 29-40.

Veatch, R. M. 1993. From forgoing life support to aid-in-dying. *Hastings Center Report* 23, 6 (Suppl.), S7-S8.

Part II, Conclusion

Barry Hoffmaster

Despite a surge of writing about pluralism, multiculturalism, and the need for cultural sensitivity, the kinds of challenges that these sorts of cultural differences pose for health care ethics and health care public policies remain vaguely and imperfectly understood. To gain a better appreciation of those challenges and how they might be addressed, at least five issues need to be examined.

The identification of cultural differences

Trying to define "culture" and subsequently to formulate criteria for distinguishing cultures and identifying sources of cultural differences are, as we saw in Part I, imposing problems. Yet the concept of culture needs to be wielded with considerable objectivity and precision, given the moral and political consequences that are now attached to it. In the deaf community, for example, there is a movement that rejects the view that deafness is a disability or a handicap in favour of regarding deaf people as a distinct subculture (Dolnick 1993). Deafness, in this view, is to be regarded along the lines of ethnicity, and deaf people are seen as constituting a linguistic minority who have their own language – American Sign Language. Feelings of "cultural solidarity", it is reported, are so strong that "many deaf parents cheer on discovering that their baby is deaf" (Dolnick 1993, 38). One moral implication of this stance is the rejection of cochlear implants as a form of treatment for children. How can the soundness of this position and the consequences derived from it be critically assessed without a firm understanding of what a culture is and why cultures are morally important?

Answering those questions is of course not the end of the matter. Suppose we adopt a crude but practical criterion that demarcates cultures along national boundaries, so that Canada, the United States, and France are regarded as having different cultures. Now the question that arises is whether any and all differences in the nature and delivery of health care in these countries are to be regarded as cultural differences. Differences in basic styles of medical practice exist in these countries. Doctors in the United States, for example, rely extensively on tests to arrive at a diagnosis, whereas physicians in Europe make more use of their clinical skills in examining patients and of the histories they obtain by talking with patients (Payer 1988). Does the mere existence of a difference between cultures make that difference cultural or must an explanation be provided to establish that it is a cultural rather than some other kind of difference? In other words, does every difference between cultures automatically count as a cultural difference? If not – if an explanation is needed – what does that explanation involve? American physicians, it has been observed, begin treatment of HIV infection with AZT earlier than French physicians, and this difference has been attributed to differences in the primary models for AIDS in the two countries (cancer in the U.S., tuberculosis in France) and to an emphasis on the concept of "terrain" in French medicine (Feldman 1992). Does such an explanation establish that the difference in treatment is indeed cultural? How are explanations of putative cultural differences to be critically assessed and validated?

In addition, when apparent differences do exist, it is not clear exactly where they originate. Even the most zealous proponents of universality recognize the existence of local differences, as an argument for the universal nature of education demonstrates:

> Education implies teaching. Teaching implies knowledge. Knowledge is truth. The truth is everywhere the same. Hence education should be everywhere the same. I do not overlook the possibilities of differences in organization, in administration, in local habits and customs. These are details. (Hutchins 1936, 66)

This is easily converted to an argument about moral education, moral teaching, moral knowledge, and moral truth. Such an argument would hold that there are universal moral truths, but would recognize that the application or interpretation of these moral truths varies in different localities and cultures. That variability would not be taken to undermine or invalidate the truth of the moral principles, however – it would simply be a matter of "detail".

The goal of maintaining hope in terminally ill patients, for example, seems to be shared across cultures and thus might be thought to be universal. Do differences with respect to disclosing information about diagnoses of terminal illnesses and bleak prognoses arise, then, because hope is interpreted differently – has different meanings – in different cultures? If so, is this a fundamental difference that invalidates the foundations of North American health care ethics, or is it merely a matter of detail?

The heterogeneity of cultural differences

There are important differences among cultural differences. When life support is stopped for a Muslim patient, for example, certain customs are supposed to be observed (Klessig 1992). When a Muslim dies, a non-Muslim is not supposed to touch the body. Health care providers could respect this custom simply by wearing gloves. Permitting family members to turn the bed so that the patient is facing Mecca at the time of death and to recite the Koran so that these are the last words the patient hears would not be unduly burdensome, either.

Sometimes the appropriate response is a compromise that involves changes on the part of both intersecting cultures. A hospital in Toronto, for example, is now offering childbirth classes to pregnant Somali women, from which men are excluded (Morrissey 1993). Fathers have become routinely involved in childbirth preparation in Canada, but the presence of men in the Somali class would, it is felt, inhibit the women. Here deviation from the established practice of childbirth preparation in Canada is necessary to counter the established male domination of Somali culture.

As these examples illustrate, some cultural beliefs and practices are patently deserving of respect and accommodation. Others, however, are controversial. Suppose an Iranian family refuses to accept a diagnosis of brain death and insists on full ventilatory support and additional aggressive procedures for their daughter (Klessig 1992). Or suppose a Chinese family insists that information about the diagnosis and prognosis be withheld from their terminally ill mother, but the health care providers feel they have a moral obligation to divulge and, moreover, can obtain informed consent to procedures only by divulging (Muller and Desmond 1992). Should the wishes of the families prevail?

Similar questions can arise for health care policies. Ronald Bayer has recently challenged what he calls the "conventional wisdom" that "acquired immuno-deficiency syndrome (AIDS) prevention programs should be culturally sensitive":

> no strategy for effective AIDS prevention can be limited by the demand that cultural barriers to behavioral change always be respected. ... The demand for cultural sensitivity in the principled and strongest sense, the sense that compels us to think carefully about the political and moral warrant for public health intervention, is ultimately incompatible with the goals of AIDS prevention. (Bayer 1994, 897)

As these diverse examples illustrate, no simple uniform response to the variety of cultural differences is plausible. But if not every cultural difference deserves deference or respect, on what grounds are distinctions to be drawn?

The connections between ethics and public policy

If it appears that respect for a cultural difference is the morally appropriate response in a given situation, does it follow that that moral position should be reflected in public policy of one sort or another? In New Jersey, for example, the law concerning determination of death contains a conscience clause that respects the religious beliefs of those who do not accept brain death (Olick 1991). The exemption is intended primarily for certain members of the Orthodox Jewish community, but also for some Native Americans and some Japanese, whose religious and cultural understandings might be violated by declarations of brain death. Most jurisdictions regard the need for a uniform standard of death as so strong that a statutory conscience clause is precluded. The approach in New Jersey has been hailed, however, as "a new direction for the development of public policy governing the declaration of death in pluralistic communities" (Olick 1991, 285). What reasons are there for establishing uniform public policies on issues of health care ethics? And when are those reasons so strong that they preclude respect for cultural differences?

The significance of variability within cultures

Virtually everyone who discusses the role of culture in health care and health care ethics emphasizes the existence of individual differences within cultures and warns against stereotyping individuals on the basis of their cultures. It has been said, for example, that "all cultures are composed of individuals and, thus, intracultural variation can be as great as, or sometimes even greater than, intercultural variation" and that "each patient must be seen as a person who has a unique belief system, with ethnic background only a part, albeit an important part, of the equation" (Klessig 1992, 316, 321). Culture does not "take" on individuals in the same way or to the same extent; the impact of culture on people is variable and unpredictable. Moreover, some individuals are exposed to multiple cultures and thus exemplify unique cultural amalgamations. What is the upshot of this individual variability for health care ethics?

The existence of cultural change

Cultures are neither monolithic nor static; they change and evolve in count- less ways, in response to countless influences. The North American practice of disclosing information to terminally ill patients has shifted dramatically over several decades and it has been proposed that the practice in Italy is shifting in the same direction for many of the same reasons (Surbone 1992). Given this dynamic, how can one take "a snapshot" of cultures and compare them to try to identify similarities and differences? Perhaps the process of change in Italy started later, is proceeding slower, or both. But if changes in the Italian approach to disclosure simply lag behind changes that have occurred in North America, in what sense are the two approaches consistent?

Health care ethics evolves, too. The strong individualism characteristic of health care ethics in North America is now being questioned by arguments for paying more attention to the interests of families (Hardwig 1990, Nelson 1992, Blustein 1993), particularly with the shift of progressively more care to the home. It is possible that the individualism of North American health care ethics will be tempered in a way that aligns it more closely with some of the central values and beliefs of cultures with which it currently seems antagonistic. Given that possibility, how can a definitive statement of the nature of North American health care ethics be formulated and used as the touchstone of moral and policy correctness in Canada? And why, then, could it not be argued that health care in North America ought to learn from the family-centred and community-centred cultures it encounters, rather than try to force those cultures to become more patient-centred?

Cultural differences are sometimes seen as deeply threatening to North American health care ethics:

> Much of modern medical practice is laced with land mines because it is predicated on the assumption that the person experiencing illness is the one to make health care decisions and who has a right, indeed almost a duty, to be told the diagnosis and prognosis. Ideas like autonomy, independence, and competence undergird communication processes and the physician–patient relationship. Serious questions can be raised about the appropriateness of

these assumptions, especially when dealing with immigrant or other groups
with cultural values vastly different from those underpinning biomedicine.
(Barker 1992, 251)

The suggestion here is that fundamental concepts of health care ethics in
North America, such as autonomy and competence, as well as the practices
that instantiate these concepts, are inappropriate in certain cultures. When
the boundaries of the self are fluid – when persons are not sharply separated
from families and communities – do individualism, respect for autonomy,
privacy, and confidentiality provide a coherent structure for understanding
moral problems in health care, let alone for resolving them?

But even if cultural differences do seem, in theory, to challenge the
foundations of Western health care ethics, when specific problems are
considered, exactly where and how that challenge arises becomes elusive. As
studies of disclosure of information to patients reveal, determining exactly
where and how cultural values are discrepant, and how the practices of
North American health care ethics might be inappropriate, is not so easy.
Comparative studies of truth-telling generally begin by observing how the
North American approach has shifted from non-disclosure to disclosure over
the past several decades and then contrast the North American practice with
continuing patterns of non-disclosure in countries such as Italy and Japan.
These studies raise some awkward questions, though. A discussion of
several cases of withholding information in Italy, for example, identifies
some of the same harms that were used to support the move to disclosure in
North America – unresolved financial problems and unsuccessful attempts to
provide for children at the time of death (Surbone 1992). But if the harms
are the same in North America and Italy, in what sense are the assumptions
behind a policy of disclosure and reasons for it in North America inappropriate for Italy?

Moreover, differences between countries could be exaggerated because
approaches to disclosure are, for the most part, described in the general
terms required by survey research. When details are added, North American
doctors seem disposed to try to obtain cues about how much patients want to
know, to tailor information to the perceived desires of patients, and to adjust
the timing of disclosure to fit patients' circumstances. In concrete terms,
then, conveying information is complex and variable, and it is not easy to
gauge how much practices in North America actually differ from practices in
other countries, particularly when what is at issue is a grim prognosis. In
Part III, Edward Keyserlingk examines this question in a comparison of the
way Native North American and European North American patients make
decisions.

In addition, when the enormous individual variability within cultures is
acknowledged, it becomes less clear that the emphasis on individualism and

autonomy in North American health care ethics is misplaced. That is so because a tempting response to that variability is to assign priority to the individual:

> To assume that a patient will react in a particular way can be as detrimental to the physician–patient relationship as ignoring the fact that differences exist among patients. Patients should always be treated as individuals first and members of a cultural group or groups second. (Klessig 1992, 316)

Why is this response not consistent with the emphasis on individualism and respect for autonomy that dominates contemporary North American health care ethics? If individual variability is ultimately more important than cultural variability, then we need to ask, again, exactly what kind of challenge do cultural differences pose for mainstream health care ethics? Others, however, such as Aboriginals, Buddhists, and Chinese would argue that collective notions of personhood that are fundamental for the traditional Aboriginal, Chinese, and Buddhist worldviews, for example, are radically different from the individualism and autonomy presupposed in much contemporary European and North American thinking. This would also hold true for most Muslims, Hindus, and Sikhs.

Thus we are left with a daunting array of questions. These questions nevertheless need to be addressed to understand the general challenges that cultural differences raise for health care ethics and how those challenges can best be met when dealing with specific moral problems or formulating public policies. These are the challenges we take up in Parts III and IV of the book.

References

Barker, J. C. 1992. Cultural diversity: Changing the context of medical practice. *Western Journal of Medicine* 157: 248-254.

Bayer, R. 1994. AIDS prevention and cultural sensitivity: Are they compatible? *American Journal of Public Health* 84: 895-897.

Blustein, J. 1993. The family in medical decisionmaking. *Hastings Center Report* 23(3): 6-13.

Dolnick, E. 1993. Deafness as culture. *The Atlantic* 272 (Sept.): 37-52.

Feldman, J. 1992. The French are different: French and American medicine in the context of AIDS. *Western Journal of Medicine* 157: 345-349.

Hardwig, J. 1990. What about the family? *Hastings Center Report* 20(2): 5-10.

Hutchins, R. M. 1936. *The higher learning in America*. New Haven: Yale University Press.

Klessig, J. 1992. The effect of values and culture in life-support decisions. *Western Journal of Medicine* 157: 316-322.

Morrissey, D. 1993. Childbirth course aimed at Somali women. *Hospital News* (Ontario) 3.

Muller, J. H. & Desmond, B. 1992. Ethical dilemmas in a cross-cultural context: A Chinese example. *Western Journal of Medicine* 157: 323-327.

Olick, R. S. 1991. Brain death, religious freedom, and public policy: New Jersey's landmark

legislative initiative. *Kennedy Institute of Ethics Journal* 1: 275-288.
Payer, L. 1988. *Medicine and culture*. New York: Henry Holt.
Surbone, A. 1992. Truth telling to the patient. *JAMA* 268: 1661-1662.

Part III

Ethical Issues in the Delivery of Health Care Services

Part III, Introduction

Michael Burgess

The chapters in Part III connect the earlier conceptual discussions with some issues that arise in the delivery of health care in biomedical institutions. These examples are selected to reflect various stages of life in which health care practitioners and members of the community are likely to encounter issues of cross-cultural health care ethics. In discussing the issues, the chapters will endeavour to represent culture as based on diversity of practices, although any discussion of practices as "cultural" will necessarily fail to represent the breadth of actual practice. Where religious beliefs seem relevant to the analysis, they will be described without any intention to suggest uniformity of practice within the religious tradition. Similarly, the discussions will attempt to articulate the assumptions underlying the health care practices but recognize that there is considerable diversity of voices within health care practice. We also take this diversity to extend to the various approaches to bioethics that are descriptive of current practices in case consultation and ethical analysis. Finally, we seek to articulate the manner in which cultural practices and assumptions of health care or biomedicine tend to limit the choice of individuals and collectives (families and communities). For example, assuming that clinical responses are required for adequate care for dying persons results in promoting a set of options that do not include non-clinical options, such as time off work for caregivers; responding to infertility with in vitro fertilization limits access for rural communities; funding traditional medicine shown effective by scientific standards assumes a specific notion of health and limits access to services that are relevant to broader notions of health. Understanding participation in health care decisions from different perspectives illuminates the role of health care practice in shaping notions of health, health care, and ethics, and how choice may thereby be limited.

Health care practitioners, families, communities, and patients often face relatively practical and sometimes urgent decisions. Standard bioethical responses, particularly those oriented to case analysis, often reinforce biomedical assumptions and power relations, despite an emphasis on the individual as autonomous (or as potentially autonomous in the case of children). Values and experiences of patients are brought into decision making about clinical services as they are relevant to determining patient interests or promoting patient autonomy. Yet patient values are rejected when they conflict with the values of preservation of the physical lives of children, protection of individualized notions of autonomy, and promoting autonomy as personal choice in the selection of effective clinical services. For instance, the appropriate use of health care services is assumed to be directed at best interests in the sense of addressing a pathological process. This will be illustrated in discussions of best interest determinations in pediatric care and end-of-life decision making for dying persons. Alternatively, people from specific heritages are sometimes uniformly characterized as different from some abstract notion of the "usual patient" in terms of how actively they wish to participate in health care decisions. This will be illustrated in a discussion of "Euro-North American" and "Aboriginal-North American" attitudes toward informed consent.

The authors necessarily bring their own assumptions to the analyses, and have tried to become aware of these assumptions through dialogue with each other. We have tried to understand how the ethical issues presented would be different if encountered in different health care systems and cultures, and to consider how the experiences might have been different had the involved parties been from a different culture. Representation of Thai culture depends heavily on accounts of the Thai authors. Descriptions and analysis of Hutterites draws on the experiences of an anthropologist author (Stephenson) and a philosopher (Burgess). The descriptions of First Nations people is based on three non-Aboriginal authors' (Keyserlingk, Rodney, and Burgess) review of the literature, the oral contributions of the team which included a person from Aboriginal heritage (Blue), and Burgess' discussion with Lesley Paulette. Representation of the Indian Hindu perspective is based on Coward's extensive personal and professional experience and scholarship in the area.

As discussed in the previous chapters, personal, cultural, and professional background is a source of assumptions that shape discussions of health, culture, and health care ethics. Although the entire project team has had the opportunity to comment on the following discussion, the primary authors and commentators have shaped the tone and direction of the analyses. The writing of academic or professional papers and the style of scholarship is not an activity with which all participants are equally comfortable.

There are two themes that run through the chapters. First, health care services and health care ethics have complex assumptions comparable to cultural background or religious traditions. The fact that the health care context and much of industrialized society share many of these assumptions makes them difficult to recognize. This is part of the reason why many people experience issues in health care ethics with a cultural dimension as a conflict between respecting the values of others and more objective notions of doing good or respecting autonomy. The apparent objectivity of these latter values is due more to the invisibility of our own assumptions, cultural or otherwise, than to their being justified as "objectively true". A careful understanding of cross-cultural dialogue must begin with the recognition of these assumptions about biomedicine and a challenging of their privileged status. Although the role of these assumptions in health care ethical and cross-cultural dialogue has been discussed in earlier chapters, these three chapters will illustrate how identification and explicit discussion enhance and improve moral discourse.

The second theme in Part III is that analyses of ethical issues in cross-cultural health care ethics must be founded on a commitment to seek and understand the full range of notions of health, meaning, and value that are assumed by all involved, irrespective of cultural or ethnic background. This theme follows from the recognition of the non-authoritative nature of our own assumptions, and the validity of the assumptions of others when considered in the context of meaning from which they arise. This too was discussed in principle in earlier chapters, and is here illustrated through specific analyses.

Chapter 10
Pediatric Care: Judgments about Best Interests
at the Onset of Life

Michael Burgess, Patricia Rodney, Harold Coward,

Pinit Ratanakul, and Khannika Suwonnakote

This chapter turns to one of the most contentious issues in pediatric ethics: parental refusal of life-saving treatment for children. Although cultural considerations enter at all levels of pediatric care, it is in the refusal of life-saving treatment that the conflict is most obvious. Refusal of life-saving blood transfusions by Jehovah's Witnesses on behalf of their children is an issue that is used in most bioethics courses and some comfort is often taken from the courts' support for saving the lives of children over protecting parents' right to express their religious beliefs in the care of their children. The usual argument is that the children are owed the opportunity to mature into autonomous individuals who can choose religious and other beliefs for themselves. But the refusal of a life-saving liver transplant for the Aboriginal or First Nations K'aila seems in some ways at odds with these sentiments and provides an opportunity to explore the role of spiritual and cultural beliefs in health care decisions for children.

K'aila was a boy born to Lesley Paulette, in a home birth assisted by K'aila's father, François, and his brother, Thaidene.[1] The first weeks of K'aila's life were clinically uneventful, except for an episode of new-born jaundice which was treated. Despite the physician's assurances, Lesley's feelings that "something was going to happen to this child" persisted.

At three months, K'aila was examined by a pediatrician. Abnormal liver function led to further tests to rule out possible diagnoses. Biliary atresia or giant-cell hepatitis were the remaining possibilities, both requiring a liver transplant. The pediatrician explained to K'aila's parents that transplantation was standard therapy with a 80–85 percent survival rate. He urged placement of K'aila on a transplant centre's active waiting list.

K'aila's parents explained their misgivings about the proposed transplant. They believed that they would be committing a "grave error if we tried to recreate our son's body". This knowledge was, according to Lesley, "manifestations of knowledge that was available to my spirit, long before it was ever available to my mind". This type of knowledge provides the basis for much of Lesley's daily activities, such as the proper disposal of hair once it has been cut from her head.

Over several months Lesley felt pressure to submit K'aila for transplantation. She and others gathered more information about the transplant, and discovered greater problems of rejection and vulnerability to infections than she had realized. She reassessed the five-year survival rate as closer to 60–65 percent. K'aila's parents informed the pediatrician that they would refuse a transplant. Since he was clearly having difficulty with their decision, they sought a second pediatrician's care for K'aila in a bordering province. The first pediatrician reported the situation to the Alberta Department of Social Services, who contacted the Department of Social Services in Saskatchewan. A court application was made requesting that K'aila be taken into custody so that the transplant could be performed without his parents' consent. Ultimately, the court denied the application for custody and upheld K'aila's parents' right to make the decision as acceptable. K'aila lived with his parents at home until his death at 11 months (Saskatchewan v. P. 1990).

Bioethical and legal analysis

The principles of bioethics can be used as a starting place to begin to specify the moral problems in the above story. Both the first pediatrician and K'aila's parents have the responsibility of seeking K'aila's best interests. The proposed liver transplant is the physician's best opportunity to avoid the harm that will befall K'aila if the liver dysfunction is allowed to take its natural course. The harms of transplant are within the profession's level of tolerance for the treatment of a life-threatening illness. K'aila's parents also have a primary responsibility to seek K'aila's benefit and avoid harm. They assess the harm of transplant to be unacceptable relative to the nature and probability of the benefit. Lesley Paulette describes this as based initially on the vision of their Aboriginal sense of spirit and then is integrated with the reason of their mind after they further assessed the effectiveness and risks of liver transplants.

The conflict, then, is about what is in K'aila's best interests, and not about whether to pursue K'aila's best interests. This could also be expressed as a conflict of authority: parental versus medical. In European and North American thought, parents' authority is usually ethically and legally based on their responsibility to care for their children, the expectation that parents love their children, and the observation that often what is in their children's best interests is also in the parents' best interests (e.g. healthy children are easier to care for). Physician authority is based on widespread acceptance that physicians have the knowledge to assess whether specific treatments are reasonable risks (i.e. that the probability and magnitude of benefit exceeds that of the probability and magnitude of harm). This situation directly opposes these two types of authority.

It is through parents' determination of what is in their children's best interests that the range of differences in family, religion, culture, and other values enter. K'aila's parents' refusal of the transplant illustrates how cultural, spiritual, and other values can enter health care decisions in pediatrics. Cultural sensitivity seems therefore to be focused on involving these values as expressed by parents in their participation in decisions about their children's health care. But there is some debate about how accommodating health professionals should be when parents' expression of cultural or spiritual values is perceived to threaten important interests of children, such as continued life.

In Canada, the legal overriding of parents' authority to determine what is in their children's' best interests is based on specific evidence that the parents are not acting in their children's best interests. In medical cases, expert testimony is sought to determine whether the care refused is required for the child's long-term well-being, and cannot be delayed without substantial risk of loss to the child. In K'aila's case, the liver transplant was the only means of preserving life, and delay meant that death would follow within the next year. The parents' refusal focused more narrowly on whether the effect of not receiving a liver transplant would be a serious breach of responsibility to K'aila. Here issues of quality of life enter the picture and the transplant specialist's picture of post-transplant quality of life contrasted with that of the Paulettes.

The Paulettes' very articulate defence of their refusal was based on both the unacceptability of the outcome and of the means to achieve the outcome. They argued that post-transplant life was potentially more a harm than a benefit. The harm they described was in part attributed to the clinical uncertainty of outcome and the effects of immunosuppressants. But another part of the harm that the Paulettes sought to avoid was the spiritual impoverishment of fighting to keep K'aila alive by "recreating him". Lesley Paulette described K'aila as a beautiful butterfly that had landed in her hands, but whose presence could only be prolonged by tightening a grip that would destroy all that was beautiful (Paulette 1993, 16). The spiritual impoverishment of the transplant was a critique of the means recommended to preserve K'aila's life. The moral harms of the transplant involved the use of another person's organ, the suppression of the body's natural rejection of the new organ, and the suffering involved in the transplant, recovery, and long-term effects of immunosuppressants. These combined to present a picture of saving life at all costs, where the Paulettes drew on their spiritual values and judged that the costs were too great.

The court sought expert testimony about the success rate and post-transplant life for infants, and agreed that current transplant technology could not provide assurance of a good quality of life post-transplant. Mr Justice Arnot seems to have recognized that K'aila's parents were clearly dedicated to K'aila. But the emphasis was on the fact that the experts disagreed. Presumably, improvement in transplant outcomes would move the court to side with undisputed medical testimony on the issue of K'aila's being deprived of a life to which he has a right, and therefore to a judgment that the parents were not acting in K'aila's interests. So the court judged that while parental authority to determine K'aila's best interests could not in this instance be challenged, the grounds for supporting the Paulettes' authority to make the judgment were that medical technology lacked adequate evidence of positive outcome. As one commentator has noted, this does not give First Nations people the legal right to use their own standard to determine either what quality of life is acceptable for their children or what methods of maintaining life violate basic notions of integrity or morality and are therefore unacceptable means by which to preserve life (Downie 1994).[2]

The basis for the judgment in K'aila's case illustrates the limitations of the expression of spiritual or cultural values through parental authority in determining children's best interests. The Paulettes were at liberty to exercise their values only to the extent that the results did not result in a harm to K'aila as defined by the courts and current medical understanding. The message about the role of cultural values in deciding children's best interests is that they are permitted to operate only in areas of medical uncertainty or inadequacy. Once advances in technology close the gap and can better manage the immunosuppression, a refusal on the same grounds as the Paulettes' is likely to be overruled unless other legal grounds are found for honouring the values that parents bring to these judgments.

In fact, the Paulettes considered whether to proceed on the basis of cultural values or their right as First Nations people under treaty to live consistent with their own cultural and spiritual values (personal communication with Lesley Paulette). They elected to challenge the medical assessment of post-transplant quality of life because that seemed the most effective means to defend their own spiritual and medical assessment of K'aila's best interest. While this means that their victory in K'aila's case is more obviously applicable to other cultural backgrounds, it also means that the established basis for challenge is medical uncertainty of outcome.

Most discussions in bioethics of parental authority to determine acceptable quality of life and means of maintaining life closely tracks this legal reasoning. As with the judgment in the Paulette case, expert medical testimony or judgment is taken as a relatively objective assessment of success rates and complications. Room for parental judgment is permitted only when there exists clinical ambiguity about outcome or where success at prolonging life is accompanied by considerable suffering. In fact, it is very rare for any medical procedure with a relatively stable outcome to be resisted as an unacceptable means; it only seems possible where, as in this case, the current medical knowledge and ability are unable to meet the burden of proof required to override parental authority.

The role of cultural and spiritual values

Cultural and spiritual values in parental decision making for children are therefore permitted only as a basis on which to choose between socially sanctioned medical procedures. Unlike the requirement of informed consent which confers a broad liberty to refuse any medical intervention in behalf of oneself, parental authority in life-threatening decisions is restricted to selecting from among a set of options which are judged to be in children's best interests. Since the courts and ethicists do not always accept medical judgments of children's best interests, the authority to make such decisions must derive from some other source. The standard according to which parental authority seems to be challenged is based on an apparent principle that it is obligatory to provide any means to salvage a child's life provided that the intervention does not also incur unacceptable suffering. Clearly the assessment of unacceptable suffering, whether in the means of prolonging life or in the resulting quality of life, requires a basis for evaluation.

Bioethics discussions often argue that the obligation to children to save their lives except in cases of extreme suffering is based on an understanding of the child as of individual moral value and yet incapable of autonomous choice. The reasons provided range from the inherent value of children, their unique individuality, parental and societal responsibility to children based on their vulnerability or on the nature of relationships, and membership in the moral community. All of these focus on children as individuals who will become autonomous and make choices based on their values. The most commonly cited ground for overriding religious refusals of treatments is that children must be given a chance to choose for themselves.

What choice are these children to make once they are autonomous? It is fallacious to think that by treating children the choice of whether or not to be treated is left for them to make once they are autonomous. The decision is made on their behalf, and they must live with the consequences of that decision and often the choices which they will have to make are shaped by the treatment decision. For example, the decision for K'aila could not be deferred until he was "autonomous". If he had received the liver transplant, his future decisions would be whether to continue with medications and perhaps whether to proceed with a kidney transplant if the medications caused renal failure. It therefore seems that the protection of children's "future choice" is oriented to protect their physical life (since they will not be able to make the choice made for them earlier), in order that they may later choose whether to share their parents' beliefs. So the choice preserved by saving life and treating against the parents' beliefs is whether to agree with the parents' beliefs. This seems a clear preferencing of the belief that physical life must be maintained despite the parents' judgment that it is against their child's best interests.

It is important to see the culturally based assumptions in these constructions of the value of children. Children appear to be valued as vulnerable beings who are potentially autonomous decision makers. Our "cultural" belief is that we must just protect children's physical lives until they develop sufficient autonomy that we cannot justify enforcing this cultural belief against their wishes. The only information relevant to decide whether or not a child ought to receive a life-saving treatment has to do with the outcome of the treatment: will the child live to enjoy the benefits of the therapy and of life? Cultural and spiritual values leading to contrary values are only permitted influence in cases of uncertainty of outcome.

The Paulettes' situation suggests that an alternative to this perspective would be to explicitly ask what the role of health care is within the parents' notion of their responsibility for their children. Hearing the Paulettes' account leaves no doubt about their love for K'aila, nor does it suggest that there is anything about the medical facts that they do not understand. It would be very difficult to make a case for any but the best of motives. The only basis for overriding their parental authority is that they have a different notion of what it is about K'aila they are to protect and nurture. Their notion of K'aila's best interests is rooted in an understanding of life, community, and nature that finds the medical interventions repugnant for their method and the predicted outcome. The court allowed the Paulettes to exercise their judgment because there was adequate medical uncertainty. But a richer notion of the role of culture in health care ethics involves allowing spiritual and cultural values to determine the role health care serves in the construction of meaning around children's roles and interests, and therefore parents' responsibilities. It is difficult to even imagine this role for cultural and spiritual values if the assumption of protecting children from physical harm as determined by objective medicine is the basis for all assessments of children's best interests.

As Lesley Paulette tells us, to understand K'aila's best interest required a careful assessment not just of his medical prognosis, but also the spiritual meaning of his existence within the context of his family and his community. Caring for K'aila's best interests meant not putting K'aila through exhaustive medical procedures for an uncertain outcome. Rather, K'aila's parents sought to strengthen his connections within his family and community for the short time before his death. Not attending to this spiritual dimension of K'aila's well-being, the pediatrician initially involved in K'aila's care did not understand the benefits and burdens of the treatment options from the Paulettes' perspective. This led to a failure in the process of informed consent – a failure that Kaufert and O'Neil have indicated is all too common when Western biomedical practices collide with First Nations beliefs and values (Kaufert and O'Neil 1990).

Towards a First Nations reading

Only one possible reading has been given to the Paulettes' story, and caution must be exercised in generalization. Lesley's own voice, which narrates K'aila's story, continuously reminds us that the beliefs and traditions of First Nations people have a great deal more to say: "As Native American people, whose cultural and spiritual traditions are steeped in a reverence for the wisdom inherent in the Creator's natural order, we felt we might be committing a grave error if we tried to recreate our son's body" (Paulette 1993, 14). Simultaneously, the Paulettes did not seek to find some ethical insight or principle that was common to all persons with their heritage. The oral transmission of wisdom through elders, coupled with the fact that First Nations cultures are diverse in their values and beliefs (Shestowsky 1993), cautions us against generalization. First Nations people "are not all the same, and their views on moral and non-moral issues are shaped by culture, geography, and different life experiences" (Elder Ron Wakagejik, cited in

Aboriginal Research Coalition 14, and reported in McDonald, Stevenson, and Cragg 1992, 3). The pediatrician sought to understand K'aila's parents and to negotiate by finding other First Nations' people who had agreed to liver transplants or who were health professionals and could explain the acceptability of transplantation from a "First Nations' perspective" ("Man Alive" show). Unfortunately, this reflects the assumption that cultural beliefs are static and homogeneous for persons with a similar heritage, an assumption that seems common to much clinical bioethics writing. But the Paulettes dealt with K'aila as a unique situation for which their responses did not in any way constrain other people of similar heritage. They were not trying to determine or discover a set of universal principles that would be applicable in similar situations, but to respond to the specific situation in a manner that was consistent with and promoted a view of the meaningfulness of their lives and that of K'aila.

The nature of harm experienced by First Nations people must be understood in terms of their beliefs in a balanced universe made up of energy fields, where the world, the environment, the community, the family, and the self are interwoven and move in harmony together. In their study, "A Lament by Women for 'The People, The Land' [Nishnawbi-Aski Nation]: An Experience of Loss", Dennis Willms and his colleagues (Willms et al. 1992) document the loss suffered by women whose northern native community becomes disrupted by the dominant Western culture (see also Anderson, Grace, Helms, James, and Rodney, in press). "The predominant component of this loss is in relations and systems of accountability; a loss of moral relations with persons, with community, and to the land" (Willms et al. 1992, 332). In other words, the harm that the dominant Western culture generated for these women went beyond the purview of Western biomedicine – that is, biological, psychological, and social "problems'. Instead, the harm was linked to the loss of the women's harmony with their community and their land. The Paulettes' experience as First Nations people illustrates how we may better appreciate Willms et al.'s (1992) warning that harm is experienced by the community and the land, not just individuals. The intervention of the Ministry of Social Services and the courts, for instance, may have affected the community within which K'aila lived. It is possible that some community members' memory of the failure to appreciate the Paulettes' spiritual concerns and the government application to apprehend will lead to a hesitancy to be candid in discussions of the role and value of children and child rearing. Health care decisions are better understood as based on the meaning that specific individuals and communities construct around caring for their children. Health or social services, courts, or ethical interventions can undermine First Nations people's trust that they will be permitted to care for their children in a manner that is based on their values and is therefore meaningful to them. Although the disrespect shown to First Nations' expression of responsibility is itself a moral harm, it also carries potentially harmful consequences of reduced effectiveness of care due to a loss of trust and candid communication.

Children's welfare from a Thai Buddhist perspective

The following is a description of how the determination of children's best interests might be considered from a Thai perspective. As discussed in previous sections, the vast majority of Thai people are Buddhist, and Thai culture has been significantly influenced by Buddhism. Yet different persons would emphasize different features of Buddhism or Thai culture, so this discussion is one of many possible perspectives. It has been developed in conversation among the Thai and Canadian colleagues and summarized by the authors. This is not an attempt to represent the full range of Thai perspectives, but to understand some elements of a Thai perspective in order to uncover our own assumptions and how they might interfere with the expression of alternative values and choices. From a practical perspective, two different angles on the issue are relevant for inter-cultural discussion. First, how would the issue of a conflict of parental and medical judgments about children's best interests arise and be managed in Thailand? Second, how does a Thai perspective help us respond to the issues in the Canadian context?

The confrontational and legal framing of the issue of determining K'aila's best interests is a reflection of the context, specifically biomedicine, bioethics, and Canadian society. This is particularly evident when we consider how such an issue might arise or be responded to in Thailand. The K'aila case is presented as an explicit conflict between parents and medical authority over K'aila's best interests, and the courts are referred to in order to determine a socially acceptable response. In Thailand, a Buddhist cultural perspective emphasizes harmony and not confrontation. It would be rare for parents to directly confront the medical interpretation, or for the courts to be involved. Even in clear cases of malpractice, the families rarely go to courts for resolution. If Thai patients or parents believe that the medical information they receive is inadequate, they are far more likely to simply go to another physician or hospital for another opinion. Since the majority of Thai people live in rural areas, they may not have recourse to another opinion unless they are willing to travel to an urban centre. Although there are public and private hospitals, treatment there is costly, so it is not uncommon for physicians to be told that the parents cannot afford the suggested medical procedure. But although Thai parents could therefore graciously take their child home and consider another opinion or seek funding for care, the Buddhist notion of compassion may be expressed by parents agreeing to any service that might cure or extend their child's life. Even procedures with significant risks might be undertaken, and then the performance of religious rituals such as merit-making (e.g. giving gifts to Monks) might be made to protect the child from such risks.

Expensive procedures such as liver transplants are difficult for any but the wealthy in Thailand to afford, but compassion plays a large role in the availability of care. Thai people perceive themselves as having many options. Physicians and hospital staff will recommend sources of charitable funding, family members will sometimes give money for medical care, monk-healers at temples offer herbal and spiritual care without charge or with a minimal fee. Thai people often respond to calls for assistance to the needy published in the popular press, and the Royal Family can often be appealed to for assistance.

The Thai family identity generally includes the parents and children as a unity of interests, although the extended family is very important, particularly in the rural areas. Although the emphasis on harmony means that parents and physicians are unlikely to have explicit disagreements over what to do for a child, Thai parents will sometimes decide that a physician is too aggressive with medical technology, and elect not to return with their child, but to see another physician, or provide care at home. In any case, it is likely that the assistance of a monk-healer will be sought for the child's welfare. The courts are not used to apprehend in any of these cases, again due to at least in part to the emphasis on harmony which avoids such a confrontational approach to managing family issues.

When children are brought home to die, the parents and family focus on providing a good death. A good death for a child is to die while being cared for by family. The Buddhist notion of rebirth supports the role of a good death as an influence in the next life. The biomedical assumption about duties to children's best interests is that duties are owed with respect to life, which ends at death. Considering the emphasis of the Thai perspective on how children's dying may have influence beyond death reminds us that the physical and objectivist view of biomedicine may well be a minority view when considered globally.

In Thailand, then, parents might be willing to accept a liver transplant if it were available for their child. Unless they were affluent, the parents and physicians would need to seek funding for the procedure and care, but there are several sources for funding, apparently as a manifestation of compassion, in Thai society. The actual transplant would likely be delayed, if it ever occurred, due to scarcity of donated livers. In the event that parents did consider the transplant to be too aggressive a response, they would likely seek assistance from another hospital or physician. If there was any need to address a disagreement with a physician, a Thai parent or patient would likely enlist the assistance of another physician or even a monk to converse about the care of their child until agreement was reached, preserving harmony.

What might be expected from Thai parents in Canada? It is important to emphasize that persons with Thai heritage will vary widely in the extent to which they think and act from the perspective of Thai Buddhism and culture. But as much as parents still practise notions of compassion and harmony, they are likely to accept a liver transplant or other medical procedures with high risk or uncertain outcomes. When they disagree with a physician, Thai parents are unlikely to directly confront the physician, but may seek the input of another physician, health professional, or perhaps a non-health professional to open the discussion in order to seek a more satisfactory response without direct confrontation. But as K'aila's parents discovered, in Canadian society physicians and provincial departments of social services are charged with the social responsibility of enforcing the morality implicit in the assumption that effective medical treatment is always in the child's interests and overrides other interests. In this context, even when the Paulettes simply withdrew from one physician and sought care in Saskatchewan, the physicians' and social services' concerns led them to seek out and confront the Paulettes. The Thai emphasis on harmony is likely to encounter similar resistance in North America.

Children's welfare from a Hindu perspective

One thing the K'aila case points out is a conflict between cultures in the ways that children's identities are understood. Whereas the doctor in the case saw K'aila as an individual child with identity and rights separate from his family, K'aila's family, consistent with their Aboriginal culture, saw K'aila's identity as sharing in the larger family "self" which extended out to include the spiritual basis of the cosmos. While the doctor sought to invoke a legal view of K'aila's "rights" as an individual child to maximize his lived time in this life, using transplanted organs and drugs as necessary, K'aila's parents saw their "obligation" in terms of safeguarding his spiritual identity which transcended this-life-only considerations. In the K'aila case we see two issues relating to self-identity in multicultural contexts and best-interest judgments on behalf of the child: (1) Is the child seen to be an "I-self" identity, having individual ethical standing from birth (or even conception) separate from the collective "we-self" identity of parents and extended family? and (2) Is the child's identity to be seen in terms of the maximum length modern medicine and technology can deliver in this physical life, or is the child to be understood as existing in a larger spiritual context which may transcend both this current life span and its physical dimension?

Many traditional cultures (and their religions) would view the child as part of the extended family "we-self" and as living a spiritual rather than a secular life. The Hindu tradition, with its South Asian cultural context, has a very strong extended family self-identity. Considerations relating to the care of the child are seen not just in terms of what is best for the individual child – although of course the individual child is important – but in terms of the child as part of the extended family and its spiritual context. It is not just the doctor and the child or the doctor and parents on behalf of the child who take decisions for the child's well-being; in an extended family, parents, grandparents, aunts and uncles, all share in the identity of the child and thus have a role to play in decision making. Nor is the child to be thought of simply in terms of this current physical life. Hinduism takes a long view with its assumption of rebirth. The current life the child is beginning is not the child's first or only life but one in a long series of lives which end in the realization of an identity with the Divine.

It must be acknowledged that there has been a gender bias in favour of sons for many centuries in the Hindu tradition and Indian culture generally. Evidence of this male child bias is found in classical Hindu scripture *Brihadaranyaka Upanisad* VI 4.20 where the parents approach sexual intercourse saying "Come, let us strive together, let us mix semen that we may have a male child" (Radhakrishnan 1968, 327). This strong preference for sons to continue the ancestral line has resulted and does result in negative judgments being made about female embryos or new-born girl babies. In the past, various rituals (e.g. the *pumsavana* in which the juice of ground banyan tree seeds is dropped by the father into the pregnant woman's nostril) were performed to effect the birth of a son. Nowadays medical technology is sometimes employed to select a male child. In such instances the "we-self" collective identity of the family may be swayed by the prospect of having to provide a large dowry (and thus deplete the family estate) and therefore opt to abort a female fetus. Here the best interests of the female fetus are clearly not being protected. In India, for example, the female–male ratio has declined from 972 females to 1000 males in 1901, to 935 females in 1981. In some sections of Hindu society female children are given less nutritious food, less medical care, and are sometimes victims of malicious neglect. While no religious or legal authority condones such wilful neglect of girl children, the right to life of at least some infant girls is in danger (Narayanan 1996, 61).

However, if one is a boy child or a girl that escapes the above bias, then the "we-self" identity can work in very positive ways. Childhood is considered sacred in many texts of the Hindu tradition. Gods and goddesses are portrayed as children as objects of spiritual devotion (e.g. the mischievous child Krishna praised in song and poem). Parents identify their children with the playful Krishna and, especially in the early years, give them their every wish. The extended family and friends take part in the naming ritual which occurs after the child is eleven days old. From six months to five years a variety of sacraments are performed to boys and girls at the most favourable astrological times for the child and the family. These rituals link the child's weal with the weal of the entire family and, through astrological synchronicity, with the whole cosmos. Weaning takes place late in the Hindu tradition and the prolonged physical intimacy between child and mother helps foster "we-self" sharing, togetherness, and ability to assimilate. Commenting on the effect of this different Indian, Hindu approach to rearing the child in its early years, Lois Murphy, a child analyst in India, writes:

> Their experience is predominantly an experience of being with the rest of the family... The constant togetherness and participation may mean that the small child is rarely exposed to new experiences without the support of a trusted person; it also provides an experience of kinesthetic and empathic richness which children brought up in cribs, playpens, carriages and other articles of furniture could not possibly have. The child comes to know and feel and intuitively to understand people with a depth grown from the time he is close to muscles and bodies (Murphy 1989).

While the "I-self" children of modern Western society grow up learning more about the mechanics of objects through the hours and days they spend taking them apart and putting them together, Indian children are given their early formation in a permissive and person-rich, indulgent environment. This changes when the child at about six years leaves the maternal world, is initiated (head shaved in sacred thread ritual), and schooling is begun. The world is then filled with obligations and the years of innocent permissiveness are over.

With this understanding of the Hindu (and Indian Christian, Jain, or Sikh) child in his or her cultural context, let us return to the questions generated by the K'aila case which were raised at the outset. It is clear that in the Indian cultural context all child rearing patterns nourish a deep "we-self" identity in the developing child up to about six years of age. From the moment of conception through birth and on to first leaving home for school, the parents and extended family see the child as an integral part of the family "we-self" sense of identity – including a built-in bias against female fetuses and girl babies. From this "we-self" perspective the child's best interests have always to be judged in the context of the best interests of the extended family. Nor is that the outside limit of the child's identity, for it is also understood to stretch out backward and forward from this physical life. The identity of the child existed prior to its current birth in countless previous lives, each filled with freely chosen actions (*karma*). The physical and psychological traces from these actions and thoughts in previous lives carry forward into the child's current life as potentialities which may promote either health or disease. Whereas the backward identity of the child with previous lives is individual in nature, the child's forward identity into future lives is both individual, if reborn as another human, but collective in nature if the spiritual goal of Hinduism – namely identity with the divine essence of the cosmos (Brahman) – is realized.

To echo the K'aila case in Hindu terms, if the parents and extended family (including a spiritual master or teacher – *guru*) judged that this child through self-discipline in previous lives had reached spiritual realization and final peace in this life, then the use of modern medical technology (e.g. liver transplant) to keep the child alive to explore its "I-self" potential (from the Western doctor's perspective) would be seen by the family and the Hindu tradition as not being in the child's best interest. Given the Hindu's view that the goal of life for all of us is, as it were, to be reborn over and over until at last we find our rest in God, one can understand the view of parents and family that perhaps the child has realized its ultimate goal of "we-self identity" with God and the cosmos and therefore no extraordinary medical measures should be used. And again, from the Hindu perspective, even if the judgment of the parents and family was wrong – i.e. on death, the child did not merge with God (*Brahman*) – the child is not ultimately lost for he or she will simply be reborn to continue forward progress via freely chosen actions and thought toward the ultimate goal – expansion of one's "we-self" to full identity with the Divine. Clearly the Hindu view in its ethical considerations transcends this current life span and its physical dimensions. But the Paulettes' experiences in caring for K'aila suggest that these values that shape Hindu views of children's best interests will only be respected in Canadian social services and courts if the parents' actual decisions either are in harmony with medical recommendations or conflict only in cases of medical uncertainty.

Conclusion

The K'aila case and the Paulettes' accounts, together with the reflections on Thai Buddhists and Indian Hindu approaches to children's interests suggest that conflict, such as the one encountered by the Paulettes, is likely in Canadian health care delivery. The conflict, however, is due as much to one set of "Canadian" cultural values as expressed in health care, social services, and the courts. These values are not "objective", but the basis on which we shape our notions of responsibility for children in the modern Western biomedical culture. Working towards an inclusive and perpetually negotiated consensus is therefore the best approach to a cross-cultural participation in pediatric health care. The first step in this dialogue is to recognize that health care, social services, the courts, and bioethics typically bring a particular "cultural" view of what constitutes being responsible for children's welfare. Conflicts with parents who do not accept the view that children's lives ought always be extended by any available means are as much a reflection of the "culture" of the health professionals and others as they are of the parents. Only open collaboration can avoid the two extremes of the moral violence of enforcing dominant notions of responsibility on the one hand and permitting clear abuse in the name of cultural sensitivity on the other (i.e. ethical relativism). By learning to be sensitive to the realities and experiences of others it should be possible to negotiate new understandings or "horizons of meaning" (Taylor 1992) in specific situations and for cross-cultural ethics in general. We can make use of rich descriptive data from anthropology and other social sciences (Lieban 1990) to inform our ongoing normative reflections (Hoffmaster 1991, 1993). The only way to avoid these problems is through genuine discussion with the goal of understanding diverse views of the value of children and child-rearing. Specific decisions about the welfare of children must take care not to enforce a particular view of children's best interests simply because it is assumed in institutional and professional practices and reflected in legal and ethical reasoning. As expressed by Sherwin, it is inappropriate to consider conflicts of parental judgment about their children's best interests under the rubric of abuse and neglect (Sherwin 1991).

Notes

1. The description of K'aila's care is based on his mother's written account (Paulette 1993), the CBC "Man Alive" video, and on the legal decision (Saskatchewan v. P. 1990), and on conversation with Lesley Paulette following her review of the manuscript for this chapter.

2. It is interesting that the Canadian Minister of Health, on the recommendations of a Royal Commission, has proposed legislation banning certain types of reproductive technology as unacceptable means of assisting the goal of reproduction. The reasons most frequently given are that the technologies violate Canadian values by commercializing and thereby commodifying reproduction. (Bill C-47; Royal Commission on New Reproductive Technologies 1993, 55-56).

References

Anderson, J. M., S. E. Grace, G. Helms, M. James, and P. Rodney. (in press). Women speaking: Heather Rose and the culture of health care. (Manuscript submitted for publication in the proceedings of "Northern Parallels: The 4th Circumpolar Universities

Co-operation Conference" at The University of Northern British Columbia.)

Bill C-47. 1996. An Act respecting human reproductive technologies and commercial transactions relating to human reproduction. The House of Commons of Canada. Second Session, thirty-fifth Parliament, 45 Elizabeth II.

Downie, J. 1994. A choice for K'aila: Child protection and First Nations children. *Alberta Health Law Report* 2: 99-120.

Hoffmaster, B. 1991. The theory and practice of applied ethics. *Dialogue* 30: 213-234.

Hoffmaster, B. 1993. Can ethnography save the life of medical ethics? In *Applied ethics: A reader*, ed. E. R. Winkler and J. R. Coombs, 366-389. Oxford: Blackwell.

Kaufert, J. M. and J. D. O'Neil. 1990. Biomedical rituals and informed consent: Native Canadians and the negotiation of clinical trust. In *Social science perspectives on medical ethics,* ed. G. Weisz , 41-63. Philadelphia: University of Pennsylvania Press.

Lieban, R. W. 1990. Medical anthropology and the comparative study of medical ethics. In *Social science perspectives on medical ethics,* ed. G. Weisz, 221-239. Philadelphia: University of Pennsylvania Press.

McDonald, M., J. T. Stevenson, and W. Cragg. 1992. Finding a balance of values: An ethical assessment of Ontario Hydro's demand/supply plan. Unpublished Report to the Aboriginal Research Coalition of Ontario.

Murphy, L. 1989. Roots of tolerance and tensions in Indian child development (as quoted by Prakash N. Desai, *Health and Medicine in the Hindu Tradition*, 26). New York: Crossroads).

Narayanan, V. 1996. Child and Family in Hinduism. In *Religious Dimensions of Child and Family Life,* ed. H. Coward and P. Cook, 53-78. Victoria: Centre for Studies in Religion and Society.

Paulette, L. 1993. A choice for K'aila. *Humane Medicine* 9: 13-17.

Radhakrishnan, S. (translator). 1968. *The principal Upanisads.* London: Allen and Unwin.

Royal Commission on New Reproductive Technologies (1993). *Proceed with care.* Volume 1.

Saskatchewan (Minister of Social Services) v. P.(F.). Dominion Law Report (69 D.L.R. 4th), 1990:134-143.

Shestowsky, B. 1993. Traditional medicine and primary health care among Canadian Aboriginal people: A discussion paper with annotated bibliography. Ottawa: Aboriginal Nurses Association of Canada.

Sherwin, S. 1991. Non-treatment and non-compliance as neglect. In *Contemporary issues in paediatric ethics* ed. M. M. Burgess and B. E. Woodrow, 71-89. Lewiston, N.Y.: The Edwin Mellin Press.

Taylor, C. 1992. *Multiculturalism and the politics of recognition.* Princeton: Princeton University Press.

Willms, D. G., P. Lange, D. Bayfield, M. Beardy, E. A. Lindsay, D. C. Cole, and N. A. Johnson. 1992. A lament by women for "The People, The Land" [Nishnawbi-Aski Nation]: An experience of loss. *Canadian Journal of Public Health* 83: 331-334.

Chapter 11
Comparing the Participation of Native North American and Euro-North American Patients in Health Care Decisions

Edward Keyserlingk

This chapter compares the relevance of the notions of autonomy, informed consent, and personal choice in the attitudes and expectations of contemporary Euro-North American patients and Native North American patients. The comparison intended is one between the two patient groups, not between two medical "systems" as such, modern biomedicine and traditional healing.[1] The specific question addressed is whether Euro-North American patients differ markedly in their views and expectations about individual autonomy, informed consent, and desired participation in health care decisions. The conclusion will be that the gap between the two patient groups in respect to these notions and expectations may be a narrow one.

This is not a claim that the specific terms "informed consent" and "autonomy" are used by both patient groups or that when they are they have identical meanings. David Schneider's observation about some other words is equally applicable to these terms which, like other notions of human agency reflecting conceptions of self and social relationships, are culturally constructed and cannot be used without qualification across cultures as if they are neutral, objective units of analysis (Schneider 1968). Terms such as "informed consent", "autonomy", and "individualism" are clearly indigenous to a Western, and more specifically Euro-North American, context. Nevertheless, in Native North American cultures there exists considerable respect for individual persons and choice. While that may be in part a result of contact with the dominant culture and modern biomedicine, these attitudes are also present in the much earlier sources of those cultures.

The conventional view – focused on idealized systems, not contemporary patients

One of the origins for a view that there is a wide gap between the expectations of the two patient groups may be the tendency in ethnographic and other studies to compare aspects of medical systems, rather than the attitudes of those availing themselves of the systems. There is no denying that significant differences exist between modern biomedicine and Native North American healing regarding, for instance, curative powers, rituals, and medicines, as well as concepts and sources of health, disease, and illness. Nevertheless, the nature of the relationship both patient groups seek with their healers and the degree of participation they want in decision making is arguably similar.

Access to patient attitudes and expectations, particularly those of Native North Americans, is obviously more difficult than is access to information about the medical systems as such. But to the extent that they are available the attitudes are arguably contextually richer and provide more reliable indicators of the distinctiveness of a culture. In this regard Marcus and Fischer (1986, 45) note that contemporary anthropologists are beginning to depend less on "their traditional media, such as public rituals, codified belief systems, and sanctioned familial or communal structures", and are resorting more to "cultural accounts of less superficial systems of meaning".

The advantages of shifting from observations about systems to the attitudes, emotions, social relationships, and expectations of people apply equally to analyses about how Euro-North American patients appear to relate to modern biomedicine. Surveys and interviews of Euro-Canadian patients regarding their attitudes and expectations about autonomy, informed consent, and choice suggest that the familiar goal of modern biomedicine as catering to fully autonomous, self-reliant, and biomedically informed patients may be unrepresentative of the actual priorities of real patients.

There is a second factor which may contribute to the conclusion that there exists a wide gulf between the views of these two patient groups. It is the fact that the two clusters of culture in question, Euro-North American and Native North American, tend to be examined in isolation one from another. Doing so is understandable since the laudable goal is to identify the distinctive features of each group of cultures and medical systems. The result, however, is less attention to the similarities and a degree of romantization of the cultures and medical systems. In reality neither culture group and neither system is static or unaffected by the other. Clearly traditional healing has been more influenced by modern biomedicine than the other way around, and it is the system most under threat. At the same time, however, modern biomedicine is also evolving. It is, for example, less resistant to holistic and alternative therapies, some features of which are central to Native healing.

Furthermore, if the focus is put not simply on users but on "contemporary" users, what must be factored into any analysis is that Native North American patients are consumers of both systems. Quah (1989) and others have observed that Native people in many countries tend to see no contradiction in seeking health care from both traditional and modern medicine. The same observation applies to Native North American patients. That should not be surprising since most Native Canadians live in or are exposed to both their own traditional cultures and those of the dominant society. In reality Native Canadian people are generally of the view that modern medical services are unevenly distributed and inadequately available to them, particularly in rural and wilderness areas. Frequent complaints are that the health care system is too complex and too often requires travel to distant towns and cities, resulting in long periods of separation from one's community. There is considerable evidence in support of those criticisms, but they clearly indicate a desire for those services.

Native people who live in or near urban settings are typically most familiar with and clients of modern biomedicine. It does not follow, however, that they have lost touch with and no longer seek help from Native healers. There is underway a rekindling of interest by Native people in traditional healing, even in large cities, and Native healers are to be found there as well. Native Canadians are at a wide variety of points on a continuum between traditional and modern medicine.

A third and related factor worth noting is that analyses of medical systems tend to be from the perspective of practitioners rather than patients. Practitioners within different medical systems, like many others who observe and comment on one or more such systems, not surprisingly find fundamental differences between "Western medicine" and "traditional medicine". There undoubtedly are such differences, particularly from the perspective of the practices, theories, and beliefs of practitioners, whether physicians practising modern biomedicine or Native healers practising traditional medicine. It is not unreasonable, however, to argue that patients who have two or more such systems available to them do not necessarily conceptualize the different therapeutic options those systems offer as choices between "alternative medical systems". From their perspective they may simply be choosing from alternative treatments (Welsch 1991; Sermsi 1989). If so, it is at least plausible that they approach these alternative treatments with similar expectations as regards, for example, the desired degree of information and participation in decision making.

Categories of disease and healing in traditional medicine

The supernatural dimension

Central to traditional Native medicine are shamans, medicine men, rituals, reliance on the spiritual power of the shaman and medicine man, spiritual guidance, belief in the supernatural etiology of some diseases, herbal and plant remedies, the centrality of the connectedness of everything in one's life, and all of it linked by a spiritual sense. The ultimate goal of medicine or healing is the restoration of the balance between all one's abilities – physical, intellectual, spiritual, and emotional.

In view of these realities it is tempting to conclude that a wide and unbridgeable gap exists between both patient groups. For Euro-North American patients, it could be said, the appropriate sentiments are confidence in scientific medicine and scientifically trained physicians, based upon full disclosure and the patient's understanding of scientific medicine. On the other hand, Native North American patients are typically characterized as having faith in the Great Spirit or Creator who gave everything on earth a unique spirit and who supports their connection, as well as faith in the spiritual guidance and powers of the traditional healer, shaman, or medicine man.

Hultkrantz (1992) has noted that, "Native American healers have paid their greatest attention to a psychosomatic medicine that is directly related to religion – a medicinal dimension largely absent among Western doctors". Observers of the interface between traditional and Western medicine in some other societies have noted that "mundane" diseases tend to be treated at home. More serious "non-supernatural" diseases (for example tuberculosis, appendicitis, serious wounds) are treated by physicians trained in Western medicine, whereas diseases thought to be supernaturally caused are attended to by Native healers (Landy 1974). Asuni (1979) observed that the Yoruba community in Nigeria have beliefs flexible enough to find harmony rather than conflict between modern and traditional medical systems. This is largely because they see different benefits in the use of each system.

Whereas modern medicine can provide a cure, only the traditional healing practice can counteract the basic cause, which could be a curse, the vengeance of a god, or the evil machinations of someone else. Once these are counteracted by traditional healing, then the curative effect of modern medicine can be effective and lasting. Similar categories appear to apply to contemporary Native North American medical beliefs and practice (Hultkrantz 1992). The etiology of diseases in the supernatural category could be attributed to a variety of causes, for example evil spirits or rule transgressions by the patient or other family members.

Customary explanations by Native healers or medicine men about traditional medicine rank physical ailments as trivial in comparison to an individual's lack of spiritual well-being (Aitkin 1990). To what extent contemporary Native North American patients agree with that ranking in theory and practice is uncertain and variable, no doubt influenced in each case by the degree and nature of each individual's contact with the dominant society in general and modern biomedicine in particular.

The herbalist dimension

Does the above sketch force a conclusion that Native and non-Native patients seek medical assistance with radically different expectations and attitudes? Not necessarily. In the first place, the two groups share the same basic motivation, the hope of a cure or alleviation, whatever the ailment and its source, as well as some degree of confidence that the traditional healer or the Western physician can help. Secondly, practitioners of both traditional and Western medicine are interested in curing and alleviating pain and illness, although neither system guarantees results.

In this regard it should be noted that Native medicine has not only a spiritualist aspect but a herbalist or plant element as well. While the two are closely intertwined in accounts of traditional medicine, Vogel (1970) and others remind us that the herbalist medicine of North American Natives can be powerfully curative due to the therapeutic properties of herbs, plants, and related compounds, independently of the spiritual beliefs, traditions, or expectations of the patients or the shamans. As Vogel demonstrates, Native medicine was very influential on Euro-North American medicine. Native herbal medicine is generally credited with being considerably more "scientific" than European medicine of the same period. Because of the ignorance and avarice of colonial physicians they were the target of considerable hostility and distrust by their contemporaries, a view shared for example by Thomas Jefferson (Vogel 1970).

Attitudes and expectations of Euro-North American patients

The endurance of faith, the recovery of holistic medicine

The depiction of the typical Euro-North American patient as insistent upon full disclosure and independent decision making, fully capable of understanding pathophysiological illness, causes, and treatment options, proves to be more a favourite construct of ethicists, lawyers, and (to a lesser extent) physicians than an accurate picture of real life patients. The religious faith factor is undoubtedly considerably diminished; trust in physicians as in other professionals has seen better days. Neither, however, is dead. Patients seeking care from scientific Western medicine appear to want more from medicine than only biomedical explanations and cures in isolation from emotional, and in some cases spiritual, implications. That health care delivery too often disappoints in these respects is not in doubt, but it arguably does so despite, not because of, patient expectations.

Despite clear indications that formal adherence to particular religions and churches has decreased, many patients and their caregivers manifest belief in a deity or spiritual powers or a sense and concern for the spiritual dimension of one's life and an appreciation of ritual. Those caring for the sick in various contexts continue to encounter some Euro-Canadian patients who believe in a deity and who, whether or not they understand the etiology of the disease, interpret illness as a form of punishment for sins and/or an opportunity for purification and the exercise of virtues such as patience, humility, or obedience. Some continue to ascribe cures to divine powers working through the physician. It is difficult to conclude that such attitudes differ substantially from, for example, an Ojibway patient who believes that her illness is the result of having broken customary laws. No claim is being made here as to percentages of Euro-North American patients who have such beliefs or attitudes. But nor is it known what percentage of Native North American patients continue to adhere to traditional beliefs and attitudes about spiritual and supernatural matters.

In view of differences in educational and professional opportunities and levels, it is undoubtedly the case that Euro-North Americans are typically more knowledgeable about science and technology than are Native North Americans. There is little doubt that Euro-North American patients typically do not share with Native North American patients to the same extent or in the same manner the latter group's traditional attitudes about the "holistic" interconnectedness of everything in life – physical, mental, emotional, and spiritual. One is therefore inclined to agree with the observation of Kaufert and O'Neil (1990, 56) who note that "Native patients may reject biomedical explanations of the pathophysiology of an illness in favour of the more holistic approaches stressing spiritual causation".

That observation, however, may also apply with some qualifications to an increasing number of Euro-North American patients. In the first place, those unfamiliar with biology, medicine, or related areas necessarily remain largely ignorant about the pathophysiology of illness and disease. Few patients have the medical knowledge to personally confirm a diagnosis or the benefits and risks of a proposed treatment. As will be indicated in a following section, for most patients trust in the knowledge, skills, and beneficence of their physicians appears to take precedence over other factors. Secondly, a growing number of Euro-North Americans subscribe to what are loosely termed "holistic" approaches to medicine and healing. Even though elements of this trend reflect little more than an interest in lean bodies, for many it reflects something deeper and more lasting. Whereas "holistic medicine" by no means implies for all a belief in spiritual causation of some illnesses, as noted above, such beliefs do persist. Alternate therapy programs, which combine for example meditation, herbal medicine, and Western therapy for a range of illnesses from hypertension to back problems, are now to be found in some clinics and hospitals (Colt and McNally 1996). The psychosomatic aspects of disease and healing are increasingly studied and validated by scientists, physicians, and patients (Moyers 1993).

It bears repeating that much of Native medicine involves little or no ritual or reference to the supernatural. The latter have received disproportionate attention in accounts of Native healing (Vogel 1970). Rituals are generally resorted to only when ordinary treatment, medications, or guidance are not successful for sick persons and a supernatural agency is suspected. Furthermore, not all such rituals are necessarily without analogies in modern biomedicine. Consider for instance what Kaufert and O'Neil (1990, 57) have remarked about consent in Native medicine and how it is linked with respect for the healer. In Native American culture, tobacco is a sacred substance given to people by the Creator to enable humans and the spiritual world to communicate. When a patient offers tobacco to a healer, "a person is demonstrating his or her respect for the healer's authority and willingness to accept the healer's advice. The tobacco offering then, is the culturally equivalent ritual to the signing of a consent form in 'White man's' medicine."

Contextual autonomy versus extreme individualism

Accounts of the attitudes of Native North American patients tend to state or imply that they put great stock in trust or faith in their traditional healers, very little in making autonomous decisions, and are generally somewhat submissive in comparison to Euro-North American patients. For example Kaufert and O'Neil (1990, 57) state that Native healers expect absolute compliance from their Native patients; the offer of tobacco means the patient will obey all instructions. They state that patients seeking a restoration of balance in their lives are expected to approach a healer with humility, sincerity, and a readiness to obey without question. By way of contrast, ethical/legal analyses, policies, and proposals have long assumed that Euro-North American patients typically do want to participate actively in their medical care, be the primary decision makers, and make fully autonomous decisions. That assumption appears to require some serious qualification.

There is considerable evidence that what this writer has called "contextual" autonomy – personal decision making which includes reference to one's familial, communal, and cultural context – is widely desired and practised even to the point of being a multicultural principle (Keyserlingk 1993b). The version of autonomy called extreme individualism or extreme rationalism is neither desired nor legitimate in the estimation of most patients. Extreme individualism is based upon what Gordon (1988, 26) refers to as the ideal modern self, one which is, "as free of traces of social and cultural determination as possible. It strives to be its own author, consciously choosing its path, able to disengage itself and step back and judge rationally what it will be, where it will go." It has a corresponding version in law, in that, "with some relatively narrow exceptions the law treats all patients and physicians the same; it posits an abstracted, objectively defined 'prudent patient' as the consumer of information and the maker of choices, and conforms all physicians' legal obligations to this uniform abstraction" (Schuck 1994, 957). Contemporary ethicists increasingly acknowledge that autonomy as extreme individualism, cut off from familial, community, and cultural settings, is distorted and destructive (Beauchamp and Childress 1983; Callahan 1984).

Some of the mechanisms made available specifically to facilitate rational and autonomous patient decision making are not in fact being used with the expected frequency despite publicity and availability. For example, in the U.S. it is estimated that the percentage of the population with advance directives is less than ten percent (Brock 1994). One of the reasons people typically give for not providing them is that they trust their family and physician to make the best decision for them at the time if they are unable to make decisions themselves (Keyserlingk 1993a). Equally interesting are some data indicating that even among those who do provide advance directives about their treatment a large percentage are prepared to allow their physician and surrogates varying degrees of leeway, from "a little" to "complete", in overriding that advance directive if the latter judge it to be in the patient's interest (Sehgal et al. 1992). It is estimated that no more than twenty percent of Americans actually sign organ donor cards. It appears that promoters of legally supported mechanisms to enable autonomous decisions may have exaggerated the demand, and that their availability has had little influence on patient attitudes or medical practice (Katz 1977).

Recent empirical research into patient preferences about being informed and participating in health care decisions is informative. Ten survey studies were examined for this chapter.[2] They have some very real limitations in that they are mainly quantitative in nature, not qualitative. What is needed is empirical research on this subject and population, with a more ethnographic and individualized focus. Nevertheless, within their somewhat limited scope they do provide some interesting and reliable data.

Most patients apparently prefer not to make medical decisions by themselves, though a minority does. Most patients have considerable trust in their physicians, both in view of their expertise and their concern for patient welfare, and trust in their family members. While almost all of them want to be informed and to participate to at least some degree in treatment decisions, many are prepared to let their physician take the major or exclusive role in treatment decisions. One study (Lidz et al. 1983) in which only 10 percent of respondents wanted an active role in decisions about their treatment, nevertheless uncovered four reasons why most patients wished to be informed: to facilitate compliance with treatment decisions, as a courtesy or sign of respect for the patient as a person, to enable a potential veto of the physician's choice or preference, to participate in the decision.

Attitudes and expectations of Native North American patients

The Native patient–Native healer relationship

No empirical research studies of the type just examined have attempted to determine the preferences of contemporary Native North American patients, as partakers of both medical systems, regarding participation in health care decisions. In this case the relevant sources available to this writer were more qualitative than quantitative and include some recent cases reported and discussed by anthropologists and others, as well as accounts by Native North American commentators about traditional beliefs and attitudes.

Native medicine does not isolate from all the other "medicinal" aspects and responsibilities of life the particular moment of coming to a healer to seek a cure. Health is a proper balance of one's mental, physical, spiritual, and emotional elements. In that context it should not surprise that the traditional patient–healer relationship and process would be highly participatory for both. Consider the following observations by an Ojibway commentator (Aitken 1990, 20):

> In our Ojibway nation, each person has always been the primary helper in his own healing process. You understood your sickness, you understood how you could get well, and you applied that knowledge. ... That means to understand that each of us is the primary and single most important person in

the healing process, the person who most needs to understand the illness and the healing process. As we look at what happens today when somebody becomes ill, it is striking that they do not know what is wrong with them. They have to go to someone who will tell them what is wrong with them. ... If we are to be helpers in our own healing process, then we need to understand sickness, we need to understand the spiritual health as well as the physical ailment and the psychological symptoms that accompany disease. ... Most importantly, in the medicine world, everything on earth including ourselves is regarded as medicinal. Everything in our being, in ourselves has a spiritual and a medicinal power.

Those observations point to a time when Native persons were expected to be knowledgeable and informed about health and illness and responsible for their health. The picture just drawn is incompatible with that of passive, submissive, uninformed patients when faced with treatment decisions. The regrets of that Ojibway commentator beginning with, "As we look at what happens today" are similar to those of Illich (1975, 90) who claimed that it was not that Western medicine turned indigenous people who were medically uninformed and non autonomous participants in their health care into now informed and responsible decision makers, but quite the opposite.

As the medical institution assumes the management of my suffering, my responsibility for my and your suffering declines. Culturally relegated, autonomous health behavior is restricted, crippled and paralyzed by the expansion of corporate health care. The effectiveness of persons and of primary groups in self care is overwhelmed by the competing industrial production of a substitute value.

But how can such accounts by the Ojibway commentator and others be reconciled with views that depict Native patients as being submissive and unquestioning with regard to Native healers? Kaufert and O'Neil (1990), for example, write that within Cree and Ojibway culture, Native healers expect "absolute compliance" from their Native patients, expect them to bring to the healing encounter a "submissive attitude", an "attitude of humility", and an acceptance "without question" of the healer's prescriptions.

Several factors may explain the apparent conflict. In the first place, as indicated earlier in this chapter, the encounter with healers for illnesses having spiritual or supernatural causes is not the whole of traditional Native medicine. The "submissive" attitude would seem particularly appropriate when the cause is a spirit and one is calling upon the mysterious powers of the healer to combat it, but less appropriate and less present when it is a question of a herbal or plant remedy known to have remedial properties. Secondly, terms such as "submissive", "humility", and "compliance" need not be viewed as negative and passive attitudes, but in this context perhaps more accurately as active and virtuous, based upon a voluntary, autonomous, and informed decision to submit oneself to the mysterious powers of the healer on the basis of faith and trust. Lastly, there are after all various forms of participation, involving more or less information and understanding. Descriptions show that some healing ceremonies and rituals require the very active involvement of the patient as instructed by the healer.

The Native patient–Western physician relationship

The apparent passivity of Native patients seeking medical assistance from Western physicians and hospitals is of course not always an indication of a relationship based on trust and faith in the physician. Nor is passivity necessarily linked in any way to a Native culture or Native attitudes as such. As Kaufert and O'Neil (1990) and others have observed, it may be involuntary passivity and submissiveness based on one or more of the following: the insensitivity of physicians and other health care providers to a Native patient's concerns and values; limited knowledge of the physician's language; the need in some cases to communicate through interpreters; socio-economic disadvantages; attitudes of resignation and alienation stemming from the historical contact with a colonial and domineering medical system; previous personal and unpleasant contacts with modern health care and paternalist health care providers; and the institutional obstacles to establishing personal and trusting relationships in hospitals and other health centres.

Some of those factors, it should be noted, also encourage passivity and discourage trusting relationships between many individual non-Native patients and physicians, but the list of hurdles is clearly longer and the hurdles higher for Native patients. That Native patients put a very high premium on trust is undisputed. It may, in view of institutional obstacles,

> be more difficult to establish personalized relationships which are considered by Native patients to be necessary to the establishment of interpersonal trust. Trust relationships in turn were felt by many Native people to be the primary feature of their consent to treatment (Kaufert and O'Neil 1990, 59).

Several reported cases provide examples of Native families and patients who wished to be fully informed and take active roles in making treatment decisions. Consider for instance the widely publicized case of K'aila, a Native infant born with abnormal liver function (Paulette 1993). The infant's physician decided that K'aila needed a liver transplant to survive and so informed his parents. The parents had serious qualms about allowing a transplant in view of their belief that it would be prohibited to recreate their infant son's body. To do so would be disrespectful to the natural order established by the Creator. In the face of considerable pressure to proceed, his parents carefully researched the medical data. They learned that the risks of rejection and infection were very serious. They decided to refuse the transplant, against the advice of a pediatrician. A court hearing was held to hear both sides and weigh the evidence. The court upheld the parental wishes, and K'aila died.

Of interest to us in this chapter is not the decision of the court, but the attitudes and actions of the parents. In view of pre-existing case law about instances where the prospects of success of a disputed intervention are very low, a court could have come to the same conclusion if the parents had been Euro-Canadians resisting the transplant on the basis of other cultural, religious, or personal values (Keyserlingk 1987). However, this case casts doubt on any suggestion that Native patients and families are always passive, compliant, and submissive in their relationships with physicians and Western medicine. This was an instance of the parents of a very sick Native North American child who clearly stated their beliefs and preferences, carefully sought out and weighed the medical data about risks, benefits, and survival rates, established a trusting relationship with one of their physicians, and held to their refusal of the transplant despite considerable institutional and legal pressure and in full knowledge that their child would die.

Another case of interest involved a Native patient referred for examination and treatment from a remote community to an urban hospital. The case is intended by the authors (Kaufert and O'Neil 1990) to illustrate, as it does, the paternalism and insensitivity too often experienced by Native patients. Of particular interest for this chapter, however, is the authors' observation (50) about consent and autonomy:

> The interpreter is using her knowledge ... to negotiate the patient's consent, but she is also using Cree models of negotiation emphasizing individual autonomy. Her final statement emphasizes her client's ultimate personal responsibility: "It's all up to you to think about".

Conclusion

The expectations of Native North American patients may not differ sig- nificantly from those of Euro-North American patients regarding trust in one's physician and the desire to be informed about and to participate in treatment decisions. That cultural factors account for some differences is undeniable. In the final analysis, however, the cultures of the two patient groups may not be as determinative of the degree of participation desired as are for instance personal preferences, the institutional context, and the amount of respect and sensitivity extended by one's physicians and other care givers.

Notes

1. By "medical system" here is intended the definition proposed by Press (1980), "a patterned, interrelated body of values and deliberate practices governed by a single paradigm of the meaning, identification, prevention and treatment of sickness".

2. See for instance: Vertinsky et al. (1974); Faden et al. (1980); Strull et al. (1984); and Degner et al. (1992).

References

Aitken, L. P. 1990. The cultural basis for Indian medicine. In *Two cultures meet: Pathways for American Indians to medicine,* ed. L. P. Aitkin and E. W. Haller, 15-40. Duluth: University of Minnesota: Garrett Park Press.

Asuni, T. 1979. Modern medicine and traditional medicine. In *African therapeutic systems,* ed. Z. A. Ademuwagun et al., 175-185. Walthan, MA: African Studies Association.

Beauchamp, T. L. and J. F. Childress, J. F. 1983. *Principles of biomedical ethics.* Oxford: Oxford University Press.

Brock, D. W. 1994. Advance directives: What is it reasonable to expect from them? *Journal of Clinical Ethics* 5, 1:57-60.

Callahan, D. 1984. Autonomy: A moral good, not a moral obsession. *Hastings Center Report,* 14, 5:40-42.

Colt, H. C. and J. McNally 1996. See me, feel me, touch me, heal me. *Life* (Sept.):34-48.

Degner, L. F. and J. A. Sloan. 1992. Decision making during serious illness: What role do patients really want to play? *Journal of Clinical Epidemiology* 45:901.

Faden, R. R., C. Becker, C. Lewis et al. 1980. Disclosure of information to patients in medical care. *Medical Care* 19:718

Gordon, D. R. 1988. Tenacious assumptions in Western medicine. In *Biomedicine Examined,* ed. M. Lock and D. Gordon, 19-56. Dordrecht: Kluwer Academic Publishers.

Hultkrantz, A. 1992. *Shamanic healing and ritual drama, health and medicine in Native North American religious traditions.* New York: Crossroad.

Illich, I. 1975. *Medical nemesis, The expropriation of health.* London: McClelland & Stewart.

Katz, J. 1977. Informed consent, A fairy tale? Law's Vision. *U. Pittsburgh L. Rev.* 39: 137.

Kaufert, J. M. and J. D. O'Neil. 1990. Biomedical rituals and informed consent. In *Social science perspectives on medical ethics,* ed. G. Weisz, 41-63. Dordrecht: Kluwer Academic Publishers.

Keyserlingk, E. W. 1987. Non-treatment in the best interests of the child: A case commentary of Couture-Jacquet v. Montreal Children's Hospital. *McGill Law Journal* 32: 413-436.

Keyserlingk, E. W. 1993a. Second generation advance directives: Will reforming the law improve the practice? *Humane Medicine* 9: 57-63.

Keyserlingk, E. W. 1993b. Ethics codes and guidelines for health care and research: Can respect for autonomy be a multi-cultural principle? In *Applied ethics,* ed. E. R. Winkler and J. R. Coombs, 390-515. Oxford: Blackwell.

Landy, D. 1974. Role adaptation: Traditional curers under the impact of Western medicine. *American Ethnologist* 1:103-127.

Lidz, C. W. et al. 1983. Barriers to informed consent. *Annals Internal Medicine* 99:23.

Moyers, B. 1993. *Healing and the mind.* New York: Doubleday.

Marcus, G. E. and M. J. Fischer. 1986. *Anthropology as cultural critique.* Chicago: University of Chicago Press.

Paulette, L. 1993. A choice for K'aila. *Humane Medicine* 9,1:13-17.

Press, J. 1980. Problems in the definition and classification of medical systems. *Social Science and Medicine* 14B:45-57.

Quah, S.R. (ed.). 1989. *The triumph of practicality, tradition and modernity in health care utilization in selected Asian countries.* Singapore: Institute of Southeast Asian Studies.

Schneider, D. 1968. *American kinship: A cultural account.* Englewood Cliffs, NJ: Prentice-Hall.

Schuck, P. H. 1994. Rethinking informed consent. *Yale Law Journal* 103:899.

Sehgal, A. et al. 1992. How strictly do dialysis patients want their advance directives followed? *JAMA* 267:59.

Sermsi, S. 1989. Utilization of traditional and modern health care services in Thailand. In *The triumph of practicality: Tradition and modernity in health care utilization in selected Asian countries,* ed. S. R. Quah, 160-179. Singapore: Institute of Southeast Asian Studies.

Strull, W. M., B. Lo, and G. Charles. 1984. Do patients want to participate in decision making? *JAMA* 252:2990

Vertinsky, I. B., W. A. Thompson, and D. Uyeno. 1974. Measuring consumer desire for participation in clinical decision making. *Health Serv. Research* 9:121.

Vogel, V. J. 1970. *American Indian medicine.* Norman, OK: University of Oklahoma Press.

Welsch, R .L. 1991. Traditional medicine and Western medical options among the Nigerum of Papua New Guinea. In *The anthropology of medicine: From culture to method,* ed. L. Romanucci-Ross, D. E. Morman, and L. R. Tancredi, 32-55. New York: Bergin & Garvey.

Chapter 12
End-of-Life Decisions: Clinical Decisions about Dying and Perspectives on Life and Death

Michael Burgess, Peter Stephenson, Pinit Ratanakul,
and Khannika Suwonnakote

This chapter applies the discussions of cross-cultural health care ethics to health care institutions' efforts to support persons in end-of-life decisions through the provision of advance directives and perhaps physician-assisted suicide. The clinical innovations of advance directives and physician-assisted suicide are based on the perspective that control over treatment decisions is one of the most important issues for persons who are dying and their care givers. This perspective on death and dying is too clinically oriented, and therefore fails to meet the immediate and pressing needs of dying persons and their care givers. The clinical approach and the ethics reflected by it can be compared to two alternative perspectives, represented in this chapter by the values expressed in Hutterian and Thai beliefs and practices. Understanding Hutterian and Thai cultural perspectives is important for mutual participation in clinical decision making because increased sensitivity will permit people of those heritages to better reflect their concerns and values in their care for dying persons. Additionally, understanding Hutterian or Thai heritage emphasizes less clinically oriented needs of all dying persons and their care givers, which may be neglected in clinical care for dying persons. Ethics discussions that are characterized by advance directives and physician-assisted suicide reflect this emphasis on autonomy in clinical decisions. Cross-cultural reflection suggests that clinical interventions must not be the sole focus of ethical judgments. Rather, ethical discourse must be treated as a means of building meaning and personal significance around experiences of death and dying. Decisions about end-of-life treatments can be considered as one means of facilitating this important social activity.

A clinical perspective on dying

Advance directives are intended to establish the limits of clinical care for patients who are terminally ill, irreversibly suffering, and who may be unable to speak on their own behalf. When medical technology and expertise can no longer offer hope of reversal of a condition that threatens life, the focus of health care shifts to palliation. Health professionals must determine the nature and extent of their responsibilities in caring for a wide range of patients whose conditions are irreversible and who often lack the competence to participate in health care decisions. The tragic circumstances of anticipating death and perhaps of reduced competence is often accompanied by pain and other discomforts that reduce the quality of life. Evaluation of when life is worth living and what palliative interventions are worth enduring requires patients' participation. Attempts to manage palliative health care must therefore find a means of engaging patients' values in the health care decisions.[1] While seeking close relatives' input is a secondary position, it is far preferable to have had definitive patient input at a time when the patient was competent. Advance directives, derived from early notions of living wills, are documents in which patients express their treatment preferences and may designate substitute decision makers (Emanuel and Emanuel 1989; Emanuel et al. 1991).

Explicitly giving patients the choice of refusing life prolonging treatment or of valuing pain relief over risk of death raises for some patients the option of requesting assistance to die sooner. Many clinicians claim that the experience of withholding or even withdrawing of treatment is dramatically different from providing the means for suicide, or actually assisting a patient to die. But from a patient perspective, there may seem to be little difference between the choice to accept the risk of earlier death in order to achieve better pain management, and the choice to accept, for example, higher levels of medication in order that death will be sooner. Some clinicians desire to be responsive to dying patients' needs and interests when there is so little that health care can actually offer. They are willing to assist patients' efforts to seek an earlier death (Caralis and Hammond 1992; Kinsella 1991).

Advance directives and assisted dying respond to the problems clinicians face when caring for these patients; these are problems with which clinicians have traditionally sought assistance from colleagues, family, friends, lawyers, courts, ethics committees, and consultants. Similarly, patients and their intimate care givers, which include family members and friends, have also been in situations where the clinical care was unsatisfactory; suffering is avoidably prolonged and aggressive care has promoted a greater magnitude or a longer period of suffering. Public and professional awareness of the high costs of care at the end of life and of cost constraints is another reason to establish patient wishes as a means of limiting unnecessary expenses without denying reasonable care. In typical bioethics language, the problem with end-of-life decisions is that it is difficult to know when the good done by prolonging life is exceeded by the harm done in prolonging the associated suffering, sometimes referred to as a conflict of beneficence and non-maleficence. This is complicated by the fact that the maintenance of persons in the last years of life accounts for a substantial portion of health care expenditures and other health care services could be more readily available if a savings were effected in end-of-life clinical care. This is often referred to as a problem of justice in the allocation of scarce resources.

Bioethics in North America promotes respect for autonomy as a key value in ethical decisions. The assessment that a life is so miserable or tragic that it is best not to prolong it is a blatant judgment of the quality of that life. Bioethics has established a tradition of giving priority to patients' own judgments about their quality of life. Beginning with research subjects' right to give fully informed consent, and extending informed consent into clinical care through shared decision making, the most recent extension of patient autonomy has been a right to refuse life-prolonging treatments. It is based on this last extension of autonomy that advance directives seek to determine what patients would want in the event of their not being able to speak for themselves and being terminally ill. The advance directive is a document that establishes one's wishes in advance of the loss of competence, and may also designate a substitute decision maker. Advance directives may also deal with topics beyond life prolonging measures, such as one's institution-alization or participation in research.

Physician-assisted suicide permits physicians (or other health profes-sionals) to provide the means for patients to take their own life when they judge that life is no longer worth living. Providing the means for a patient to commit suicide takes autonomy one step further than deciding in advance of one's incompetence what life prolonging measures to accept or refuse. In the case of assisted suicide, autonomy is not simply a basis for determining which of the available clinical services should be used to prolong life. Physician-assisted suicide is based on the claim that terminally ill patients' judgments about their quality of life can justify physicians acting definitively to end life. This is usually justified on one or both of two arguments. (1) Autonomy of patients includes a "right to die" and fairness or justice requires that patients who are incapable of acting to end their own lives are owed assistance to fulfil their wishes. (2) There is no morally relevant distinction between "letting die" and "killing", so the justification of one counts for both.

Advance directives and assisted dying characterize a relatively pervasive clinical perspective on death and dying that is focused on end-of-life decision making about clinical services. There are reasons for the emphasis on these particular decisions over others that arise in experiences of death and dying. One reason is that despite a recent trend to palliation in homes, hospices, and palliative care units, death is, in North America, largely institutionalized as a medical event.

The focus on end-of-life clinical decisions is also influenced by the tendency in health care to adhere to doctrines of "scientific care" and of "consistency as justice". Both of these doctrines suggest that similar clinical cases ought to receive similar clinical care. This is proposed as scientifically sound because the indication for treatments is a scientifically understood pathological process that is repeated in patients who have the same condition. A simple notion of justice is that persons with similar needs ought to receive similar resources, and in health care this translates as providing the same clinical resources for those patients with the same clinical condition. Ideally, for every clinical condition there is a standard of care that reflects the current scientific and clinical experience. Patients who refuse the standard of care seem to be requesting unscientific or unfair treatment.[2]

Bioethics and the philosophy of medicine make sense of patients' requests not by challenging the doctrines of scientific standards of care and notions of justice, but by emphasizing that patients' autonomous choices must be respected. The result is that caring for dying patients is focused on determining their wishes regarding clinical options. So exceptions to the "clinical standard of care" for a particular condition must be justified by documenting patients' autonomous wishes. Aberrant requests, such as for assisted dying, must further be maintained as anomalous, or else they will become the standard of care for all patients in similar clinical states. The family communication in clinical settings will often focus on issues such as what is "best" for dying loved ones as patients (i.e. as recipients of health care), what would or do they want, and are they competent to make these decisions.

A third reason for the focus on clinical decisions has to do with the gate-keeping function of health professionals. Simply put, the gate-keeping function of physicians is intended to limit access to potentially harmful substances and procedures to those instances where there is good chance that the benefits will outweigh the harms. This widely accepted role of physicians is one of the reasons that they are so attractive as the gate-keepers for assisted dying. But physicians also have the cultural authority to define when access to health care services is justified, and often to decide when it is covered by insurance plans. Physicians are persons from whom access must be gained, but also from whom permission must be sought for exceptions to the standard of practice. Physicians document the basis for their treatment recommendations, for future reference in caring for the patient and as protection in the event of litigation. Deviation from the standard of care is also documented for similar reasons. Advance directives are one means of documenting refusals of the standard of care, both to guide future care and for legal defence.

One final reason for the focus on end-of-life clinical decisions is rooted in the fact that the costs of caring during the last years of life are widely publicized and characterized as a waste of public resources. Since bioethics reflects health care's focus on the responsibility of health professionals to protect the rights of patients, there are only two acceptable means of reducing expenses that are "wasted" on people who are dying. The first is to determine that for particular patients specific services are "futile", and therefore carry no significant sense of benefit that is denied that patient when the service is not offered. The second is through determining that particular patients have made autonomous decisions not to receive specific services. Both advance directives and assisted dying limit the use of clinical service by providing opportunities for patients to reject service and achieve savings in an area of perceived waste.

We turn now to perspectives on death and dying that are different from the clinical perspective described above which can meaningfully affect health care decision making. There are at least two ways of understanding how a diversity of views might affect care for dying persons. One understanding would be the classic bioethics view that diverse views can be expressed through the exercise of individual autonomy by patients and substitute decision makers who participate in determining health care for specific individuals. For example, some individuals may find organ transplantations objectionable as a means of prolonging life and specifically refuse that intervention. The specific patient or familial perspective is therefore brought to bear on the clinical decision. Another understanding of how diverse perspectives affect care giving for dying patients is that people operate from a background that includes the social and spiritual meaning of death and dying. The influence of a diversity of views can then be understood as patients' and families' attempts to locate clinical decisions within that context. For example, the refusal of an organ donation in the K'aila case discussed earlier was based on a rich worldview about bodily integrity, relationships with nature, and the value of life. An implication of this more complex understanding is that bioethics and the delivery of clinical services must serve the construction of meaning within broader cultural and spiritual contexts, instead of viewing them as obstructions to clinical care that have legitimate expression only as they influence autonomous treatment decisions. The following discussion of the social and spiritual significance of death and dying will further develop the theme of locating health care decisions in this culturally rich context.

Cultural perspectives and informed consent

Through advance directives or their substitute decision makers, patients can bring their personal values to bear on health care decisions. Religious perspectives that insist nothing be done to shorten life can be expressed as strongly as individuals wish through these mechanisms. Individualized expressions are preferable to general characterizations for identifiable groups. For instance, Jehovah's Witnesses who refuse blood must do so personally, and health professionals ought not assume that the every Jehovah's Witness will refuse blood transfusions. Health professionals have the responsibility to listen carefully to each individual patient and family in order to assist them to make health care decisions that are consistent with their values and life goals.

The choice to accept or forgo life sustaining treatment reflects deeply personal and socially rooted values about spirituality, quality of life, and responsibility to self and others. Arguments that the treatments could not reverse the terminal condition or third party assessments that the quality of life is or is not worth sustaining are not adequate to override autonomous consent. Similarly, autonomous decisions to refuse treatments ought to be respected independent of arguments about the effectiveness of the treatments or the high quality of life after treatment. So values, whether cultural, religious, or other, can limit the care that one receives or be the basis for an insistence on treatment that prolongs life.

The emphasis on patient autonomy as expressed through advance directives or proxy consents does not guarantee accurate or current expression of patient preferences regarding the use of life-prolonging measures (Danis et al. 1994; Emanuel et al. 1994). This is due to a definition of "effectiveness" as reversal of a pathological process. Health professionals report frustration with patients or families who insist on expensive palliation or life-prolonging treatments in irreversible conditions. The tendency to deny the position that autonomy justifies health care system costs for end-of-life decisions is reflected in the literature on futility (Schneiderman et al. 1990; Brett and McCullough 1986; Waisel and Truog 1995; Murphy 1988). This emphasis on the (wasted) costs of preserving life that will never be self-sustaining shapes the clinical and legal standards of care. Concerns about cost-effectiveness drive the basis of the standard of care from determination of effectiveness, or risk–benefit ratio, to a cost–benefit judgment that the specific service is a poor use of resources unless the service will either reverse the pathological process or significantly alter the prognosis. The judgment that a service is poor in terms of this cost–benefit analysis will sometimes be taken as justification to withhold on the basis of a "medical decision" (palliative care is a major exception, and there is likely significant variation between clinicians and institutions). The route of autonomous expression of personal values in clinical decisions as a point of entry for spiritually or culturally based values is therefore inadequate for even the decision to use or forgo life saving treatments. This is primarily because the options are limited by a notion of benefit that is defined by the clinicians' and institutions' "cultural" value: cost-effective reversal of a pathological process. The influence of patients' or families' cultural values is thereby restricted to decisions among services valued and offered on the basis of the values assumed by the clinicians.

In fact, the best route for cultural and spiritual values to be integrated into health care decisions is through understanding clinical services as serving the broader goals of meaningful death and dying. Services that are poor cost-effective means of reversing a pathological process may be relevant to a "good death" for other reasons. Replacing the original question of how to accommodate cultural values in health care decision making, the cultural perspective asks what role health care serves in the construction of meaning in death and dying. Determining the role of health care service in this broader goal requires the participation of patients and families in specific cases and involvement of a diversity of cultural perspectives in policy discussions.

Social and spiritual significance of death and dying

The clinical perspective is characterized above as an impoverished approach for the construction of meaning in death and dying. The focus on clinical services over social dimensions has been discussed elsewhere as a process of medicalization, where a physical condition or deviant behaviour initially considered to be an individual misfortune or a community nuisance is conceptualized as a diagnosed condition with recommended treatment procedures, and the dedication of social resources for research into causes and treatment. Jana Sawicki, writing about new reproductive technologies, describes a common use of "medicalization" as follows:

> The term "medicalization" usually implies the negative phenomenon of reducing political, personal and social issues to medical problems thereby giving scientific experts the power to "solve" them within the constraints of medical practice. (Sawicki 1991, 119)

Medicalization of dying through the clinical focus sustains a view of suffering, dying, and intimate care giving as private (Burgess 1994). The medicalization of dying extends to advance directives and assisted dying which continue to focus attention and social resources on clinical responses and away from the more socially and personally important features of death and dying. But dying, life while dying, and life while one is of diminished competence are social events that have effects on the community. Family and friends who may be intimate care givers (Jones 1984; 1992; Koopman-Boyden 1979; Brody 1976; Zarit 1985), as well as staff of health care facilities or residences are among those directly affected. Co-workers, clients, and friends of those delivering personal or professional care are less directly, but often profoundly, affected. These persons and relationships are the social resources upon which the dying person must draw to define meaning and quality of life during incompetence and dying. But the same persons and relationships have social, vocational, and domestic respon-sibilities to fulfil. Yet there are few provisions for adjustment of these responsibilities. The workplace demands are constant, as are the domestic. Social activities which may be important for emotional stability during times of intense care giving are likely the first to be sacrificed by care givers (Jones et al. 1992). The focus on increasing patient and/or proxy par-ticipation in establishing sensitive clinical care dedicates social resources to the clinical elements of incompetence, suffering, and care giving. Less "institutional" responses might make available paid time off for care giving, flexibility in work hours, job security, and publicly funded or community based assistance in vocational and domestic duties to enable care giving and respite. But social resources are primarily directed to providing clinical services and options (Azzarto 1986; Binney et al. 1990).

These social arrangements reflect cultural and spiritual values that are reinforced through the institutions of health care, work, and domestic responsibility. If participation in health care decision making is limited to expressing cultural and spiritual values in selecting options within clinical care, then it is not a surprise that the so-called integration is unsatisfactory. The issue of whether pain management or life extension is a higher priority may seem insignificant to a dying person who is trying to make sense of the end of life in terms of accomplishments, spiritual goals, memories, and relationships. To some people, clinical decisions may play important roles in constructing the meaning of their death and life, while for others they may be a distraction, or a means of pursuing more important goals. The next sections provide examples of these experiences and their insights for the role of cultural values in health care decisions.

Religious ethics and secular ethics

Jeffrey Stout, in his book *Ethics After Babel*, suggests that the contemporary language of morals in theological and philosophical debate have been unnecessarily impoverished by attempts to use only broadly applicable notions of ethics (Stout 1988). Stout argues that both "secular" ethics and moral reflections within particular religious traditions have opted to gain widespread credibility. This has been accomplished by limiting the language and scope of moral discourse in a manner that ignores much of what is reasonably considered moral terrain. Stout uses the example of "moral abomination", suggesting that if it were reintroduced into moral discourse it would express the moral sentiment of revulsion in reaction to moral atrocities. Stout's example illustrates how the use of religious and theological discourse enriches "secular" moral discourse by providing language and concepts that more completely describe moral experience. Similarly, reflection on different cultural and religious communities may reveal moral sacrifices and values inherent in the evolution of society. Only by understanding specific experiences of the meaning of death and dying is it possible to begin to shape the goals that clinical services must serve in order to be sensitive to cultural and spiritual values.

Hutterian dying

In separate projects in rural southern Alberta, Stephenson and Burgess have been struck by the ability of some persons to better adjust their lives to accommodate the opportunity to care for dying persons. In southeastern Alberta, it seemed that the Hutterians, some Natives, and some of the local ranching families were able to better accommodate dying persons. They were often (though not always) able to accommodate chronically ill and sometimes disabled persons. Stephenson's work on the Hutterian colonies in southern Alberta provides a more detailed look at Hutterian death experiences and treatment of the disabled. (Stephenson 1984; 1985).

The tragic death of one member of an Alberta colony revealed how a quick death deprived the members of the colony of the opportunity to care, to organize social events around their member's dying and death, and for the individual to work through spiritual and social issues. It is revealing to note that this quick death with reduced physical suffering would have been relatively ideal in the wider society, but for the Hutterians it was particularly difficult. Very different attitudes towards pain and suffering, the individual, and social obligation are manifested by the Hutterians and the culture that surrounds them. This is, of course, bound up in a way of living and a belief system that gives purpose and meaning to dying and suffering as intrinsic parts of living itself. Three relevant themes are the emphasis on community, agrarian life, and dying as valued in the religious community.

The Hutterian way of life has always emphasized community as the primary value in organizing social life, historically shaped by persecution and immigration to avoid oppression. Part of the basis for their coherence as a group and for their being persecuted has to do with their specific religious beliefs and how they choose to live according to them. So the whole notion of being a group which survives together and is "in but not of the world" likely contributes to the solidarity of the community. The Hutterians see themselves as a perpetuation of the communal lives of the apostles (Acts II) and the adult baptized members of each communal farm are the reborn body of Christ himself. We have witnessed examples in southern Alberta of young Hutterian men who temporarily work outside of the colony, but do not choose to leave it permanently. It is in this social, spiritual, and historical context that the care of dying persons fits into a way of life that gives caring for dying persons its particular meaning in the community.

Hutterian vocational life has maintained an agrarian approach to producing the material necessities. This may mean the latest technologies are adopted towards farming, but many roles overlap or are interchangeable. Young men work as assistants in various farm enterprises prior to settling into one as a primary occupational role. Young women work in gardens, the communal kitchen, in the kindergarten, and at all manner of painting and cleaning as well as child care. This facilitates the valuing and accomplishment of caring for dying persons by sustaining vocational roles that are largely interchangeable, allowing co-operative interchange of roles as needed. Specifically, as members are needed for important tasks of caring, others are adequately skilled to fill in for them. Similarly, when caring for a family member reduces the available time for domestic duties, others supply food and fill in other tasks. Further, the social roles of all members of the colony enable some sharing of the caring tasks, permitting important respite to the care givers. In economic terms, none of this reduces the ability of families to cope with the loss of income that greatly distorts caring behaviour in the wider society. The Hutterians are communal and all persons have equal material benefits from the labour of the group.

Death and dying in a Hutterian community is a valued element of social life – indeed of living itself. The final days of life are intensely social and expand the social interaction and numbers of people on a colony. Stephenson even postulates that the social activity characteristic of dying may benefit Hutterian women who are socially isolated around the ages of 55–60, and that this may contribute to earlier death than for the general population (Stephenson 1985). It is during gathering for the dying and death of community members that some courting takes place. Children and distant relatives visit the dying person, with as many as 500 persons attending the funeral. Support for the dying person, care givers, and the fulfilling of domestic and vocational chores are common features of the community's life. The routine integration of caring for dying persons and of dying persons themselves into the community is an indication of the value placed on dying and caring for dying persons.

For the Hutterians the value of caring for dying persons is an important element of community life that reflects their historical–social–spiritual context, and their vocational and domestic role flexibility. What would participation in health care decision making at the end of life look like if it were directed to these goals?

Cultural sensitivity to Hutterians would involve recognizing that health care services are a means of achieving not clinical–scientific goals but spiritual and community based goals. Setting aside for the moment the problem of enforcing a general cultural picture on individuals, the goals of clinical services would be to return the dying person to the community, to enable an enduring and conscious participation in the community's activities around care giving, and arranging the various activities that surround care giving and community. To accept this as the goal of clinical care then permits the specific patient and family groups to negotiate decisions about clinical care which best serve these goals. Rather than offering clinical options for their efficacy or because it is standard of care, the relevant clinical options become those that serve the goals that the patient and care givers use to make the experience meaningful.

Cultural sensitivity to Hutterians in end-of-life decision making then implies that clinical services are seen as serving the promotion of meaning in the sense of participating in the social activities that are part of the patient's heritage. But it also means that Hutterian patients' autonomy must be respected in their selection of how the clinical services are in fact used, and which goals they actually elect to pursue. For many Hutterians, this decision will be made in a social context, with significant demands made by the community. But to treat this as inadequately autonomous is to enforce a standard of autonomy developed in the clinical setting to protect individuals from the power of physicians. Such a standard is inappropriate for the influence of family and community members of Hutterian communities who are less isolated in their sense of self and the meaning they bring to dying.

A Thai perspective on dying

The Thai approach to caring for dying persons is best understood as a range of practices that are rooted in Thai cultural values and Buddhism. The cultural values of harmony and gratitude are important to understanding caring for dying persons. The notion of harmonious relationships is expressed among the four elements (i.e. earth, water, wind, fire) within the body and between the mental and physical elements of the human system, between the self and others in interpersonal relationships, and between the self and the natural environment. Confrontation is to be avoided in interpersonal relationships as a kind of violence that disrupts harmony. This may limit the extent to which explicit disagreements about patient care will arise.

The value of gratitude is based on the recognition that we owe debts to parents, relatives, teachers, friends, and any person who has helped us along our way in life. In the case of parents, we are also obligated to repay them, for example by taking care of them, when needed, by whatever means is within our power. This is particularly necessary when parents are vulnerable to suffering or dying. Thus suffering or dying parents in Thai culture are likely to receive considerable care from their children.

Buddhism is the cornerstone of Thai culture. Its concepts, ideas, and values have much influence on the way Thai people think and act in matters relating to life, illness, and death. The value of compassion and the notion of *kamma* are central to Thai Buddhism.

The value of compassion is the central teaching of Buddhism (see chapters 2 and 7). Different forms of compassion are found in interpersonal relationships among Thai people. In these relationships compassion usually means to have a sympathetic understanding of others, a willingness to prevent harm to them, and to alleviate their suffering as well as not to increase it. In the case of Buddhist monks, compassion is manifested in selfless work to relieve and alleviate suffering of people caused by illness and disability.

Buddhism emphasizes *kamma* or a principle of retribution as deeds and their consequences, or causes and effects (see chapter 2 for detailed explanation). We are the sum of our deeds. Good deeds bring good results (effects) and bad deeds bring bad consequences. This belief in the importance of *kamma* is associated with the belief in merit-making and rebirth. In Buddhism, life is a process of causes–effects (i.e. interwoven activities) and it is a beginningless and endless process. What we call "life", "birth", and "death" are only integral parts in this endless process (called the "wheel of life", or the round of existence). Rebirth is the repetition of birth (arising) and death (passing away) and the quality of rebirth depends on the quality of life at present. The continuity and duration of life and death for each individual is incalculable. If the collection of bones of one person's repeated rebirths were amassed, they would form a mountain of skeletons. The imprisonment in this life process of birth, death, and rebirth is the result of one's own deeds, good or bad. It is within our power to either remain in the cycle (process) or to escape from it. Merit-making is an important means, and a necessary one, to ensure a good rebirth. In this connection, Buddhist monks are regarded as a "field of merit" in which lay people can cultivate good *kamma*. Offering foods and necessities to monks is one way of merit-making. In the case of dying, this kind of merit-making is believed to be a necessary way for the dying person to accumulate merit in the last stage of life to ensure a good rebirth and/or to mitigate bad *kamma* in the past. The practice of meditation is another kind of merit-making to instil wholesome states in the mind of the dying to ensure a good rebirth (see discussion of this in chapter 7).

In the care of dying persons, the Buddhist notion of compassion is particularly important, as is the notion of a good death. A good death might be considered one in which the person receives the best physical and spiritual care. Physical care pertains to medical treatments, nursing care, and herbalist treatments that may comfort or even extend life and maintain mental lucidity. Spiritual care involves inviting a Buddhist monk to visit and instruct the dying persons in meditation in order to instil positive mental states which will affect how the person is reborn. The monk's visit will focus the dying person's mind on their good deeds, as well as provide an opportunity for the dying person to "do merit-making".

In most cases people are cared for at home by their family. Generally, the family is willing to care for the dying person, in part because of the Buddhist notion of compassion. Gratitude is an element of Thai culture that is the basis for a duty to care for parents that is apparently contested by some Thai people, particularly some members of the younger generation who sometimes view gratitude as a way to impose parents' values and perspectives on their children.

Not all dying people are cared for at home. Some Thai people require hospitalization for treatment, in which case the patients and family are responsible for costs. Thai people have alternatives, however, due to the responsiveness of the public and the royal family to appeals for assistance, and the options of public and private hospitals and Buddhist temples. For example, AIDS patients may be initially cared for by their families. The patient's or family's embarrassment, however, may encourage the consideration of other alternatives. Many AIDS patients are cared for in a

Buddhist temple. The Buddhist monks are supported by donations from the community, and the monks provide lodging, food, and herbal medicine and teach meditation. Meditation is also believed to have physical effects such as the lengthening of life, through the influence of a better mental life. Dying persons are also given tasks or chores for the temple, with the belief that by contributing to the community the person will feel better and not useless or focus only on death. The temple provides a support group or community for dying persons for the sake of their mental health. The maintenance of a "wholesome mental state", including hope, is supported by these activities. The Buddhist notion of *kamma* suggests that the disease is a combination of *kamma* cause and physical cause, so maintaining a wholesome mental state is not only a spiritual focus. Since one cannot know how soon the influence of bad *kamma* will be exhausted, it is possible that hope is not unreasonable (i.e. that the negative *kamma* will be exhausted and permit physical treatment to be effective). It is not uncommon for persons at temples to live longer than is expected given their physical illness.

Families are often supported by extended family members when they are caring for dying family members. Relatives in rural areas might send money to assist with the costs of caring and other family members may take turns providing care and keeping company with the dying person. While there is not a government subsidy for time off to care for family members, it is not uncommon for immediate family members to take time off of work in order to care for the dying person. The ability to take time off, or to hire additional assistance for care giving is obviously dependent upon economic status. As a result of this difference for the care giving of dying patients, the Thai government is under increasing pressure to provide increased resources for dying persons, particularly for those who are poor, or located in urban areas. Many of the monks work to exhaustion in the temples caring for dying persons, thereby relieving the government of the responsibility to provide or support services for the dying.

There are people in Thailand who are concerned that some Thai physicians trained in the Western methods of medicine might enforce a medical model and discredit traditional medicine by promoting the notion that modern biomedicine can solve all the problems of life. Traditional medicine is more likely to be thought of as one means of addressing health and spiritual concerns, as illustrated by the belief that there is both a *kamma* cause and a physical cause to illness, and that both causes ought to be addressed.

The exercise of autonomy in health care decisions through informed consent is insufficiently compatible with respect for Thai culture and Buddhism. Thai culture and Buddhism suggest that clinical services are a set of reasonable responses to the physical dimensions of illness and dying, but that issues directly relevant to death and rebirth are more important. Clinical options that might not be offered, such as prolonging life without reversing the pathological process, can be important to enable the dying person a visit from the monk for meditation and merit-making. Palliative services might be refused on the patients' behalf by family because it clouds patients' minds and ability to meditate. The goal must not be to merely understand how Thai culture and Buddhism might lead to different clinical services, but rather how clinical services might serve the goals of Thai culture and Buddhism for dying persons.

Conclusion

Participation of people from diverse cultural backgrounds in end-of-life decisions must begin with the recognition that the meaning of death and dying is always rooted in a historical–social–spiritual context. Cultural sensitivity begins with the recognition that everyone, including health professionals and ethicists, operates from a perspective and that those perspectives are valid ways of constructing meaning around death and dying. It is inadequate to offer patient participation in clinical decisions about which services to receive. Rather, cultural sensitivity comes from first asking what particular activities and issues are important for the dying person and the care givers. Then the clinical options that enable participation in these meaning building activities can constitute the appropriate care for the particular situation. Only sustained commitment to valuing care giving and dying in the context of patients' own experiences will adequately respect death and dying as part of our diverse social and spiritual community.

We can learn from the above examples how dying and care giving for dying persons is embedded in a context that itself must be served by the clinical options. Hutterian dying is embedded in a context of family and Hutterian community, and Thai dying is located in a strong familial care giving and Buddhist notions of compassion, supported by care that is available through visiting monks or at temples. These different approaches to dying are different from the focus on end-of-life decision making in many biomedical and bioethics discussions in at least two ways. First, dying is perceived to be a passing on to another state of life and care giving is tied to notions of honouring the person and the passing. Second, the emphasis on the roles of family, community, and religion in dying provides a context for the dying persons and the care givers to shape the meaning of both dying and care giving.

These are points of contrast with a bioethical obsession with promoting autonomy in the determination of what clinical services the dying person wants. The emphasis in biomedicine on clinical interventions requires specialized knowledge and delivery by health professionals. Historically concurrent is the growth of the biotechnology and pharmaceutical industries. These forces create a very expensive health care system that has recently become an ineffective and expensive system of care for dying persons. But the costs of health care has combined with other features of industrialized life to increase the cost of living and made it difficult to afford time off from vocational duties to care for dying persons at home. Care giving for dying persons is either a professional responsibility, or one that is performed by those who can most easily be spared from duties related to income (i.e. those with the lowest income, often women). The shift of care for the dying to the home attempts to redistribute the costs of expensive and ineffective use of health care resources without restoring the economic and social or religious factors that support familial and community care giving for dying persons in more traditional societies.

It is also worrisome to ponder whether biomedicine and biotechnology will eventually undermine the meaning of dying and caring for dying persons in traditional communities such as Thai or Hutterian, as well as what may be a preferable distribution of responsibilities for caring for dying persons. Perhaps it would be better if we learned from other cultures how to shape for ourselves a social approach to dying that better integrated care giving and honoured dying persons rather than debating between professionalizing and ghettoizing their care, while preserving a sense that we have done all that could be done based on "objective" scientific medicine.

Notes

1. The term "patient" is used throughout this chapter to refer to people who are in the role of receiving health care services, and therefore for whom clinicians assume responsibility for their welfare and autonomy.

2. This is not to deny that much current clinical teaching includes understanding patient perspective and the role of social and psychological influences on illness. But even historical analyses of this development acknowledge the tendency to listen primarily for the signs of underlying pathology (cf. Armstrong 1984).

References

Armstrong, D. 1984. The patient's view. *Social Science and Medicine* 18:737-744.
Azzarto, J. 1986. Medicalization of the problems of the elderly. *Health Social Work* 11:189-95.
Brett, A. S. and L. B. McCullough. 1986. When patients request specific interventions: Defining the limits of the physician's obligations. *New England Journal of Medicine* 315:1347-1351.
Brody, E. M. 1976. Women in the middle and family help and older people. *Gerontologist* 21:471-81.

Burgess, M. M. 1994. The medicalization of dying. *Journal of Medicine and Philosophy* 18:269-279.

Binney, E. A., C. L. Estes, and S. R. Ingman. 1990. Medicalization, public policy and the elderly: Social services in jeopardy? *Social Science and Medicine* 30:761-771.

Caralis, P. V. and J. S. Hammond. 1992. Attitudes of medical students, housestaff, and faculty physicians toward euthanasia and termination of life-sustaining treatment. *Critical Care Medicine* 20:683-60.

Danis, M., J. Garett, R. Harris, and D. L. Patrick. 1994. Stability of choices about life-sustaining treatments. *Annals of Internal Medicine* 120:567-73.

Emanuel, L. L., E. J. Emanuel, J. D. Stoekle, L. R. Hummel, and M. J. Barry. 1994. Advance directives: Stability of patients' treatment choices. *Archives of Internal Medicine* 154:209-73.

Emanuel, L. L. and E. J. Emanuel. 1989. The medical directive: A new comprehensive advance care document. *Journal of the American Medical Association* 261:3288-3293.

Emanuel, L. L., M. J. Barry, J. D. Stoeckle, L. M. Ettelson, and E. J. Emanuel. 1991. Advance directives for medical care: A case for greater use. *New England Journal of Medicine* 324:889-95.

Jones, D. A. and N. J. Vetter. 1984. A survey of those who care for the elderly at home: Their problems and their needs. *Social Science and Medicine* 19:511-14

Jones, D .A. and T. O. Peters. 1992. Caring for elderly dependants: Effects on the carers' quality of life. *Age and Aging* 21:421-428.

Kinsella, T. D. 1991. Will euthanasia kill medicine? *Annals of the Royal College of Physicians and Surgeons of Canada* 24:489-492.

Koopman-Boyden, P. G. 1979. Problems arising from supporting the elderly at home. *New Zealand Medical Journal* 4:282-86.

Murphy, D. J. 1988. Do-not-resuscitate orders: Time for reappraisal in long-term care institutions. *Journal of the American Medical Association* 260:2098-2101.

Sawicki, J. 1991. *Disciplining Foucault: Feminism, power, and the body.* New York: Routledge.

Schniederman, L. J., N. S. Jecker, and A. R. Jonsen. 1990. Medical futility: Its meaning and ethical implications. *Annals of Internal Medicine* 112:949-954.

Stephenson, P. H. 1983-1984. "He died too quick!" The process of dying in a Hutterian colony. *OMEGA* 14:127-134.

Stephenson, P. H. 1985. Gender, aging, and mortality in Hutterite society: A critique of the doctrine of specific etiology. *Medical Anthropology (Fall)*, 356-363.

Stout, J. 1988. *Ethics after Babel: The languages of morals and their discontents.* Boston: Beacon Press.

Weisel, D. B. and R. D. Truog. 1995. The cardiopulmonary resuscitation-not-indicated order: Futility revisited. *Annals of Internal Medicine* 122:304-308.

Zarit, S. H., N. K. Orr, and J. M. Zarit. 1985. *The hidden victims of Alzheimer's disease: Families under stress.* New York: New York University Press.

Part III, Conclusion

Michael Burgess

Cultural background contributes to the meanings of various activities and roles. Participation in health care by any patient or family member ought to be focused on how clinical services serve these meanings. Part III has discussed examples of how health care services might serve meaning in the context of birth and caring for children, informed consent, and in dying and caring for dying persons. Issues are often presented as cultural conflicts because some set of culturally related beliefs or goals appear to interfere with patients' or family's understanding of the purpose or effects of health care services. This characterization of a cultural conflict assumes that there is no cultural context implicit in the purpose for which the clinicians might intend the service (e.g. palliation, reversal of a pathological condition, or prevention). Recognizing the assumptions in health care delivery that help form the meaning of health care delivery for clinicians and others who are involved identifies the influence of these assumptions on assessments of the moral nature of the service (e.g. the liver transplant for K'aila) or the weighing of the outcome (e.g. pain management for some Hutterites). Additionally, too heavy an emphasis on differences between cultures can result in generalized descriptions of "other cultures" that are bereft of case-specific context. These descriptions may be as oppressive as ignoring difference (e.g. the characterization of Aboriginal North Americans as more oriented to trust and compliance and less on participation in health care decisions). Much of cross-cultural ethics seems to suffer from this "fallacy of detachable cultural descriptions" which characterize cultural elements as generalizable and static (Rubinstein 1992).

Part III has been very limited in terms of the range of ethical issues considered, its limitation to cases and not policy, and the range of cultural heritages discussed. It would clearly not be possible to be comprehensive in terms of the range of perspectives within a single cultural heritage, much less to include a wide range of perspectives. The main point from these considerations is how to identify and recognize our own cultural perspective (including seeing biomedicine as a culture) through understanding other perspectives. The first step in understanding each new perspective is to consider what issues are relevant for the patient and family's construction of meaning and how that might affect the clinical support and services.

Although the range of issues discussed has been very limited, the general lesson for case analysis is that participation in decisions and in patient care must always consider the social context in which the patient and all involved relatives and friends are struggling to find and create meaning. Conflicts or even different perspectives without conflict are not merely differences in patient and family perspectives, but also stem from the meaning that health professionals (and ethicists) seek to find in their own participation. It is a manifestation of the power and perhaps lack of self-awareness of health care personnel when they are able to ignore their own struggle with the personal and social meaning of their actions and represent it as objective and scientific medicine (i.e. biomedical culture) while judging other perspectives as failing to understand. At the case level, the beginning of successful negotiation of cultural diversity in health care delivery is recognizing that we are all trying to find meaning in the activities, and to find ways to understand each other and how the health care services may be provided in a manner supportive of constructing diverse meanings.

Although the policy level will be discussed in Part IV, two lessons from this section are instructive. First, policy discussions of "cultural" differences in participation in health care cannot work from abstracted notions of different cultures, but must aim at community participation that is sufficiently diverse to represent a wide range of practice. Second, policies directed at cultural sensitivity must begin by recognizing that for individuals, families, and communities the goals of health care services may be much broader than restoring and protecting a narrow definition of physical and emotional health. Serious efforts to assist persons from diverse cultural backgrounds to find meaning in the care of their children, their sick, and their dying may often mean that health care services must be used quite differently, may be refused, or that services not typically thought of as related to health (e.g. social services, religious services, or community support) may be more relevant than some health services.

To conclude, it seems that the critical question to ask when faced with an ethical issue in health care delivery that appears to have a cultural component is, "What am I assuming about this situation in order to make it meaningful to me, and how are the patient and family different in their need for meaning?" Explicitly identifying that one is working from a perspective and is open to accommodate others' perspectives reduces the power imbalance in health care delivery and provides at least an opportunity for dialogue. Dialogue can lead to mutual construction of multiple meanings that are far richer for all involved than the approach in health law and ethics which tends to focus on determining which perspective is authoritative. Whether health care institutions and other contexts of delivery can be sufficiently humane and flexible to permit this negotiation is an issue taken up in the following section (Part IV).

Reference

Rubinstein, R. A. 1992. Culture and negotiation. In *The struggle for peace: Israelis and Palestinians,* ed. E. W. Fernea and M. E. Hocking, 116-129. Austin: University of Texas Press.

Part IV

Health Policy: A Cross-Cultural Dialogue

Part IV, Introduction

Patricia Rodney

In Part III, it was argued that health care services and health care ethics have complex internal assumptions that are often taken for granted. In other words, those of us delivering health care and debating its ethics are as embedded in our culture as those who are the recipients. The authors in Part III therefore claimed that successful negotiation of health care delivery begins when we recognize the diverse meanings that we all – patients, professionals, ethicists, and so on – bring to the clinical encounter. The same can be said for health policy development and implementation.

As was articulated in the Conclusion of Part III, health policy must aim for public participation that is sufficiently diverse to represent a wide range of meanings. Moreover, health policy must not limit its attention to dominant (Western biomedical) views of health and health care delivery. Yet health policy itself is a westernized notion; it arises from Western institutional and political structures. Overcoming the biases that this creates will take some critical self-reflection on the part of those who develop and implement health policy. The chapters in Part IV have been constructed with this requirement in mind. Although the chapter authors acknowledge that by addressing health policy per se we are commencing from a Western perspective, we have attempted to ameliorate this by bringing our voices together to speak from our own diverse cultural standpoints and individual meanings. Blue, Keyserlingk, Rodney, and Starzomki start off in chapter 13 in a spirit of self-reflection by offering a critical look at North American health policy. Chapters 14 and 15 point to health policy issues in largely uncharted territory. Hui and Tangkanasingh explore modern biomedical threats to Chinese herbology and traditional Thai medicine in chapter 14. And in chapter 15, Glickman sheds light on the ethical implications of the "greening" of conventional medicine. Thus, as the chapters unfold we broaden our view from predominantly North American contexts to international and global health policy concerns.

The latter feature is consequential. Western health policy has traditionally been concerned with the allocation of resources for health care, and unfortunately less concerned with resources for health. As the authors of a comprehensive empirical review of the determinants of health of populations have warned:

> The ways in which society regulates employment and economic cycles, provides education, assists its members in times of economic or other difficulties, sets up strategies to counteract poverty, crime, and drug abuse and to stimulate economic and social growth have just as much, if not more, impact on health than do the quantity and quality of resources being invested in the detection and care of illness. (Renaud 1994, 318)

What this means is that health is not only embedded in diverse cultural meanings (as was seen in Parts I and II) but is also closely tied to economic, social, and political conditions. Given the emergence of an increasingly global economy, where capital flows around the world to serve the interests of an economically dominant elite (Laxer 1996, 22), attending to health policy at international and global levels as well as local and national levels is essential. The authors hope that what we have articulated in our chapters will generate more thought and more work in health policy development and implementation at all four levels. While the issues covered in Part IV are not exhaustive, we believe that they are instructive.

References

Laxer, J. 1996. *In search of a new left: Canadian politics after the neoconservative assault.* Toronto, Canada: Viking.

Renaud, M. 1994. The future: Hygeia versus Panakeia?. In *Why are some people healthy and others not? The determinants of health of populations,* ed. R. G. Evans, M .L. Barer, and T. R. Marmor, 317-334. Hawthorne, USA: Aldine de Gruyter.

Chapter 13
A Critical View of North American Health Policy

Arthur Blue, Edward Keyserlingk, Patricia Rodney,
and Rosalie Starzomski

In this chapter, the authors explicate a number of issues in North American health policy. First, the various forms of health policy are explored, with a discussion of the limitations of North America's predominantly legalistic approach. Next, the authors address a number of systemic inequities in the application of health policy. Public participation in health policy is often posited as a means of reducing such inequities, and so the authors conclude this chapter by exploring some of the promises and limitations of public participation.

The critical view of North American health policy that the authors put forward in this chapter is timely. Canadian and American health care systems are undergoing substantial reform at an unprecedented rate (Christensen 1995; Storch and Meilicke 1994). This reform is directed at improving cost containment as well as the quality of care delivered, although it has been weighted significantly on the former (Council on Ethical and Judicial Affairs, American Medical Association 1995; Lamb and Deber

1992). In fact, cost containment has escalated to the extent that a number of observers (on both sides of the border) are warning that the foundations of health care and patient/professional relationships are in jeopardy (Evans 1992; Iglehart 1994; LaPuma 1994; Mariner 1995; Mohr and Mahon 1996; Phillips and Benner 1994; Rachlis and Kushner 1994; Scanlon 1996/1997; Shindul-Rothschild et al. 1996; Sibbald 1997; Wolf 1994). This means that critical self-reflection on the part of those who develop and implement North American health policy is particularly urgent.

Various forms of health policy

Within Canada and the United States, policy takes a variety of forms. These forms include personal ethics, common customary or traditional practice, guidelines, international human rights and health-related legislation and agreements, decisions by courts, provincial and federal health related statutes and regulations, various provisions of the Charter of Rights and Freedoms, some provisions and sanctions of the Criminal Code, and (in Quebec) a variety of health related sections of the Civil Code.

Strictly speaking, the first and least intrusive policy vehicle/level is that of no (formal) policy at all, in deference to practice, custom, or tradition. Interestingly, this is an option not always given sufficient consideration once a health related problem is identified and a lack of relevant policy is alleged.

Guidelines comprise a more formal step on the policy ladder, though typically without clear or onerous sanctions if they are not followed. They can be institutional (e.g. a hospital's "Do Not Resuscitate" [DNR] guidelines), or professional (e.g. a health profession's Code of Ethics), or national (e.g. research guidelines). Guidelines may also be "quasi-legal" in nature, as may become the case with the directives on ethical research from the Canadian Tri-Council Committee.

Whereas decisions by courts are in the first instance meant to determine blame and provide compensation in particular disputes, in effect and in the aggregate they also establish on an on-going basis – by establishing precedents – a large portion of prevailing health policies. Such decisions include, for example, informed consent, medical negligence, confidentiality, treatment refusal, and so forth. Recourse to the law in one form or another for health and other matters is a peculiarly Western, and more specifically North American, approach. Many other societies rely far more on custom, tradition, and shared expectations, which to varying extents serve analogous roles to those of law in North America and Western Europe.

Recourse to the law as a form of North American health policy has several explanations. These include the prevailing social and legal tradition giving pre-eminence to individual rights, the culturally pluralist history and composition of North America (with subsequent resort to law and legislation as a means of ensuring minimum standards of practice and compensation for a society of widely divergent views and values), and the fact that health care (at least in Canada) is seen as a public good for the state to regulate and distribute.

The choice of the best policy vehicle for a real or alleged health related problem or danger supposedly amenable to policy formulation is often assumed to be self-evident in a society prone to concluding about all problems that "there ought to be a law". In fact, it is seldom evident and requires careful attention. Good health policy creation or reform would seem to call for consideration of at least the following in choosing a specific type of policy: i) the seriousness and scope of the alleged problem; ii) the goal to be realized; and iii) the most effective and least intrusive means of realizing the desired goal. In some cases the "no formal policy" approach will or should be judged the most appropriate. In some cases the alleged problem is not serious enough or widespread enough to justify the curtailment of choice and use of policy making and enforcement resources. "Mediating" structures or groups closer to the problem and solution such as families, communities, churches, or particular professions/disciplines providing the technology or service in question may be the best locales to make the value and other choices involved.

One of the now standard mechanisms for making decisions about health policy levels and content in Western pluralist and democratic societies is that of assigning at least the preliminary role to groups mandated by agencies, professions, or legislatures. They may well be the best vehicles available for weighing and representing all the sides and implications of the health matter under consideration. However, given their pluralist composition and the high priority given to consensus seeking, one of their serious and well documented limitations is the tendency to select the moral "middle ground" and implicitly thereby promote the status quo in their choices of policy levels and content (Neville 1979; Walters 1987). This is not surprising, considering the conflicting views and values in the larger society for which and to which these commissions speak. Later in this chapter, the authors' discussion of the Oregon experience illustrates such a limitation in action.

While the choice of one or another form of law as the appropriate policy level for a health related matter is sometimes justified, there are dangers and limits to be considered in view of the unique context and characteristics comprising health care delivery. The ultimate concern of legal policies, whether courts or statute law, is that of rights. Rights are clearly often at issue in the health care context, all the more so in the impersonal cultural contexts of large institutions where the individual patient is likely to be treated as a stranger by strangers. However, a rights focus implies and fosters an impersonal context and a relationship of adversaries – one claiming a right, the other denying a duty. In reality, a group of adversaries disputing rights is a limited and distorted picture of what in most cases is at issue. For this reason the legal policy response is often an inadequate vehicle to address the larger picture in which needs are as important as rights and interests, in which an ethics of responsibility encompasses far more than claiming rights and giving rights, and in which the health professional– patient relationship should ideally be built on trust and dialogue rather than on the minimal requirements of the law (Keyserlingk 1981). While legal policies ensuring respect for rights are in large part made necessary by the impersonal cultural contexts in which much of health care is delivered, excessive recourse to such rights based legal policies risks taking that setting for granted and perpetuating it, rather than transcending and challenging it.

Systemic inequities

At the same time that much contemporary North American health policy takes for granted the culture within which it is located, the implementation of health policy (in all its forms) betrays a number of systemic inequities. One source of these inequities is geographic. This is particularly evident in problems with the distribution of health care in rural and isolated regions of Canada.

The distribution of health care services within the Canadian system is achieved through a process of regionalization. This process distributes three levels of services – tertiary, secondary, and primary. In tertiary centres, a broad scope of services is accessible because of widespread availability of medical specialists and technology (for example, cardiac care programs). In secondary centres, fewer medical specialists are available, while in primary settings, neither medical specialists nor technology is readily available. Thus citizens of major urban centres often have the best available high-technology services and medical specialists, while citizens of isolated and rural areas may see less specialized professionals and providers. When referrals are made from primary to tertiary centres for specialized services, patients and their family members may expend large sums of money and suffer the social and psychological consequences of being away from family and community when they are most vulnerable. Moreover, while all three levels have health care professionals and providers to offer supportive treatment and care to patients and families (for example, community care workers, family physicians, nurses, and social workers), supportive treatment and care is often thinly spread in isolated and rural areas such as the Canadian north.

In remote northern areas of Canada, the population receives most of its health care from community care workers, nurses, and social workers, while physicians, psychologists, and other professionals/providers are not available for more specialized medical treatment. Physicians should be included in all levels of service, including primary care (Gutkin 1996). Equally, primary mental health care should include those with the skills and knowledge to provide comprehensive psychological service – psychologists. However, the health policy imposed by provincial and national governments in Canada means that professionals such as psychologists and physicians are not readily accessible for people in rural and isolated communities. Indeed, in a recent study of the supply and utilization of physicians completed by the Manitoba Centre for Health Policy and Evaluation, Roos (1996) found not a shortage but a problem of distribution of physicians in Manitoba. The same distribution problem exists with other doctorally prepared specialists. For instance, the Canadian Registrar of Health Service Providers lists 75 doctoral level psychologists in Manitoba, with 69 located in the city of Winnipeg and only 6 serving the rest of the province. The maldistribution of medical specialists creates a systemic inequity whereby individuals who live in Winnipeg receive a level of treatment not available to those who live in rural and isolated regions.

This inequity is also reflected in the distribution of disease and disorder among the isolated rural populations. The 1996 Roos report indicates that there is no question but that this affects rural and northern First Nations populations in particular. Manitoba spends almost 50 percent more on a Winnipeg child than it does on one living in the north, despite higher needs in the north. Manitoba spends 34 percent more on an adult living in Winnipeg than it does on one living in the rural south, despite rather equal needs in these populations (Roos). The government, however, continues to allocate more rather than less of the health care budget to the southern population centre. Ruth Wilson and her colleagues (1994) have recently demonstrated similar inequities in relation to renal dialysis. They examined the effects of relocation of a group of First Nations people (Cree) for dialysis treatment. They found that the relocation affected not only the individual patient but also the family and the community. The data indicate that end-stage renal disease is 2.4 to 4 times more prevalent in First Nations populations than the nation as a whole. First Nations people are much more likely to have diabetes and those with diabetes are twice as likely to progress to end-stage renal disease. While there is adequate equipment and specialists for dialysis throughout southern Ontario, only now is there consideration of placing a satellite dialysis system where First Nations people living in a rural area can have better access.

Arguments have been made that other development is more critical in northern areas and that health care should take second place to community development. Many of the northern areas still lack adequate sewage disposal, clean drinking water, roads, schools, and the other necessities of life readily available in the southern areas of Canada. However, health policy makers should not trade off one for the other; both health care and community development need immediate attention.

Thus, despite Canada's explicit commitment to universal access to health services, it seems that there is a disjuncture between what is promised and what is actually received. As the situation in Manitoba illustrates, and as Stephenson's chapter 5 reminded us, First Nations peoples are at a particular disadvantage.

A second (and not unrelated) source of systemic inequities in North American health policy implementation can be found at the intersections of gender, race, and class. That is, women, people who are homosexual, people of colour, people who have recently immigrated to North America, people with disabilities or chronic illnesses, and/or people living on the socio-economic margins of society do not have the same opportunities to access effective health care services as their more advantaged counterparts (Anderson et al. 1997; Cassidy et al 1995; Sherwin 1992; Thorne 1993). Yet the social determinants of their health (Renaud 1994) mean that they are in more need of health care.

There is substantial empirical evidence of systemic inequities at the intersections of gender, race, and class – evidence that is well portrayed in chapters 4 and 5 of this volume. Other sources illustrate a plethora of inequities. For instance, research shows the burdens of home care on women (Bunting 1992), the exploitation of impoverished women in surrogate motherhood contracts (Royal Commission on New Reproductive Technologies 1993), the poor treatment of patients with mental health problems (Mohr and Mahon 1996), the inadequate care of the elderly in nursing homes (Oberle and Grant 1994) and acute care hospitals (Rodney 1997), and widespread racial and ethnic disparities in American health care delivery (Watson 1994).

Systemic inequities in health care, whether related to geography, or to the intersections of gender, race, and class, or both, raise important questions about whose voices are being heard in the development and implementation of health policy. Currently, such questions are being taken up in debates about public participation in health policy decision making.

Public participation?

Most reports dealing with public participation in health care decision making propose that public participation is a good thing and that it leads to more equitable decision making in health policy. However, there is little empirical evidence to support this claim (Charles and DeMaio 1993; Starzomski

1997). Research has been constrained because there is little consensus or conceptual clarity about what the terms lay, consumer, community, public, or citizen participation actually mean. This lack of clarity has led to the development of analytic frameworks that outline various levels of public participation, helping to establish that public participation is not a homogenous concept (Arnstein 1969; Charles and DeMaio).

A number of potential benefits have been claimed as a result of public participation in health care. These benefits include defining the needs of the community, developing effective ways to meet those needs, fostering a sense of civic responsibility, and promoting a sense of belonging to a community. Furthermore, there is potential for an enhanced level of concern for fellow citizens, a greater sensitivity to the social causes of many health problems, and sensitivity to the needs of different ethnocultural groups (Centre for Health Economics and Policy Analysis 1991; Charles and DeMaio 1993; Checkoway 1981; O'Neill 1992; Reiser 1992; Starzomski 1997; Wachter 1992).

Despite such benefits, some significant concerns have been raised about public participation in health care policy making (Starzomski 1997). Lay involvement may encourage interest group politics and decision making based on emotional or personal responses rather than on facts and input from those with expertise. Health care professionals/providers and bureaucrats who prefer to retain centralized power are worried that their power base may be eroded (O'Neill 1992). Conversely, there are concerns that in some cases public participation may consolidate the power of bureaucrats rather than the community groups they are charged to represent. Furthermore, there may be a move to emphasize majoritarian decision making to the detriment of disenfranchised groups. Finally, the process may be slower if there is public consultation about issues (Centre for Health Economics and Policy Analysis 1991; Charles and DeMaio 1993; Checkoway 1981; Reiser 1992).

There are a few examples in the literature where attempts have been made to involve the public in health policy decision making. In Canada, discussions have taken place at the Royal Commission level and through a national forum (National Forum on Health 1997). In several provinces, there have been recent major efforts to include citizens as those provinces reform their health care systems (British Columbia Ministry of Health 1991; 1993; Centre for Health Economics and Policy Analysis 1991; Nova Scotia Government 1994). However, the outcome of these efforts is still unclear.

In the U.S., particularly in Oregon, discussions at the grassroots level have been occurring about how health care resources should be allocated (Dougherty 1991; Jennings 1988). The social experiment that occurred in Oregon shed light on a number of areas about public involvement in health care decision making. In an attempt to deal with the rationing questions that had been plaguing the state, elected officials, "consumers", and health care professionals/providers attempted to define an adequate minimum standard of health care for their citizens (Nelson and Drought 1992; Oregon Department of Human Resources 1992). This was a process whereby Oregonians sought to discover whether they shared a tradition of values that would help them define which package of health services constituted the common good. Proponents of the Oregon plan praised its boldness and suggested that it would bring discussions of appropriate care to the forefront so that the issues could be debated in the public arena. Opponents suggested that the voices of the Medicaid patients, who were having their care rationed, were not heard in the debate, and that the plan discriminated against poor women and children. Opponents also illustrated many of the problems that arise when using quality of life indicators as a means of determining how resources should be allocated (Eddy 1991; Fox and Leichter 1991; Garland 1992; Golenski and Thompson 1991; McPherson 1991; Menzel 1992; Veatch 1991).

The process used in Oregon illustrated that the task of prioritizing health services involved a judgment based on facts and values, requiring the incorporation of public values about the health care system, with ethical, economic, and outcome approaches to policy decision making. Despite the efforts of many researchers, there are still uncertainties about how society might use outcome data to set priorities. Although the idea of determining health outcomes, ascertaining how people feel about those outcomes, and then giving priority to treatments that produce more preferred outcomes sounds simple, it is fraught with complications. Not the least of these complications is major methodological concern about the current methods used to measure outcomes (Hadorn 1991; 1992; 1993).

In summary, in both the United States and Canada there is a need to conduct research about the role of the public in health care, and to determine at what level of the system the public should be involved. In Canada, there are currently no examples where public opinion and community values about health care priorities have been determined to the same extent as in Oregon. And the American experience in Oregon was not unproblematic. Together, the magnitude of current cost constraint measures, the preponderance of rights based legal policies, and the systemic inequities in the implementation of health policy point to the need for all North Americans – members of the public, professionals/providers, ethicists, policy makers, and so on – to engage in a more thoughtful moral discourse about health care priority setting and reform.

References

Anderson, J. M., I. Dyck, and Lynam, J. 1997. Health care professionals and women speaking: Constraints in everyday life and the management of chronic illness. *Health* 1(1):57-80.

Arnstein, S. 1969. A ladder of citizen participation. *Journal of the American Institute of Planners* 25:216-224.

British Columbia Ministry of Health. 1991. Closer to home: The report of the British Columbia Royal Commission on Health Care and Costs. Victoria: British Columbia Ministry of Health.

British Columbia Ministry of Health. 1993. *New directions for a healthy British Columbia.* Victoria: British Columbia Ministry of Health.

Bunting, S. M. 1992. Eve's legacy: An analysis of family caregiving from a feminist perspective. In *Critique, resistance, and action: Working papers in the politics of nursing,* ed. J. L. Thompson, D. G. Allen, and L. Rodrigues-Fishcr, 53-68. New York: National League for Nursing Press.

Cassidy, B., R. Lord, and N. Mandell. 1995. Silenced and forgotten women: Race, poverty, and disability. In *Feminist issues: Race, class, and sexuality,* ed. N. Mandell, 32-66. Scarborough, Canada: Prentice Hall Canada.

Center for Health Economics and Policy Analysis. 1991. *Summary report: Health care and the public: Roles, expectations and contributions* (Fourth Annual Health Policy Conference). Hamilton: McMaster University Center for Health Economics and Policy Analysis.

Charles, C. and S. DeMaio. 1993. Lay participation in health care decision making: A conceptual framework. *Journal of Health Politics, Policy and Law* 18 (4): 883-904.

Checkoway, B. 1981. *Citizens and health care: participation and planning for social change.* Toronto: Pergamon Press.

Christensen, K. T. 1995. Ethically important distinctions among managed care organizations. *Journal of Law, Medicine and Ethics* 23 (3):223-229.

Council on Ethical and Judicial Affairs, American Medical Association. 1995. Ethical issues in managed care. *JAMA* 273 (4):330-335.

Dougherty, C. J. 1991. Setting health care priorities: Oregon's next steps. *Hastings Center Report,* 21(3):1-10.

Eddy, D. 1991. Oregon's methods: Did cost-effectiveness analysis fail? *JAMA* 266(15): 2135-2141.

Evans, R. G. 1992. U.S. influences on Canada: Can we prevent the spread of Kuru? In *Restructuring Canada's health services system: How do we get there from here? Proceedings of the fourth Canadian Conference on Health Economics,* ed. R. B. Deber and G. G. Thompson, 143-148. Toronto, Canada: University of Toronto Press.

Fox, D. and H. Leichter. 1991. Rationing care in Oregon: The new accountability. *Health Affairs* 10(2):7-27.

Garland, M. 1992. Justice, politics and community: Expanding access and rationing health services in Oregon. *Law, Medicine and Health Care* 20(1-2):67-81.

Golenski, J. and S. Thompson. 1991. A history of Oregon's basic health services act: An insider's account. *QRB* 17(5):144-149.

Gutkin, C. 1996. Vital signs. *Can Fam Physician* 42:1864.

Hadorn, D. 1991. The Oregon priority-setting exercise: Quality of life and public policy. *Hastings Center Report* 21(3):11-16.

Hadorn, D. 1992. The problem of discrimination in health care priority setting. *JAMA*

268(11):1454-1459.

Hadorn, D. 1993. *Outcomes management and resource allocation: How should quality of life be measured?* (Health Policy Research Unit Discussion Paper Series: 93:7D). Vancouver: University of British Columbia.

Iglehart, J. K. 1994. Health policy report: Physicians and the growth of managed care. *New England Journal of Medicine* 331 (17):1167-1171.

Keyserlingk, E. 1981. Law, ethics and biomedicine: Towards a healthier interaction. *McGill Law Journal* 26:1020-1035.

Jennings, B. 1988. A grassroots movement in bioethics. *Hastings Center Report*, 18(3 [supplement]):1-16.

Lamb, M. and R. B. Deber. 1992. Managed care: What is it, and can it be applied to Canada? In *Restructuring Canada's health services system: How do we get there from here? Proceedings of the fourth Canadian Conference on Health Economics,* ed. R. B. Deber and G. G. Thompson, 159-164. Toronto, Canada: University of Toronto Press.

LaPuma, J. 1994. Anticipated changes in the doctor-patient relationship in the managed care and managed competition of the Health Security Act of 1993. *Arch Fam Med* 3:665-671.

Mariner, W. K. 1995. Business vs. medical ethics: conflicting standards for managed care. *Journal of Law, Medicine and Ethics* 23 (3):236-246.

McPherson, A. 1991. The Oregon plan: Rationing in a rational society. *Canadian Medical Association Journal* 145(11):1444-1445.

Menzel, P. 1992. Oregon's denial: Disabilities and quality of life. *Hastings Center Report* 22(6):21-25.

Mohr, W. K. and M. M. Mahon. 1996. Dirty hands: The underside of marketplace health care. *Advances in Nursing Science* 19 (1), 28-37.

National Forum on Health. 1997. *Canada health action: Building on the legacy* (Vol 1 and 2). Ottawa: National Forum on Health.

Nelson, R. and T. Drought. 1992. Justice and the moral acceptability of rationing medical care: The Oregon experiment. *Journal of Medicine and Philosophy* 17(1):97-117.

Neville R. 1979. On the National Commission: A Puritan critique of consensus ethics. *Hastings Center Report* 9 (2):22-26.

Nova Scotia Government. 1994. *Nova Scotia's blueprint for health care reform.* Halifax: Nova Scotia Government.

Oberle, K. and N. Grant. 1994. Results of the AARN initiative regarding the impact of health care cuts. (unpublished research report). Edmonton, Alberta, Canada: Alberta Association of Registered Nurses.

O'Neill. M. 1992. Community participation in Quebec's health system: A strategy to curtail community empowerment. *International Journal of Health Services* 22(2):287-301.

Oregon Department of Human Resources. 1992. *The Oregon health plan.* Salem: Oregon Department of Human Resources.

Phillips, S. S. and P. Benner, P. 1994. Preface. In *The crisis of care: Affirming and restoring caring practices in the helping professions,* ed. S. S. Phillips and P. Benner, vii-xi. Washington, DC: Georgetown University Press.

Rachlis, M. and C. Kushner. 1994. *Strong medicine: How to save Canada's health care system.* Toronto, Canada: Harper Collins.

Reiser, S. 1992. Consumer competence and the reform of American health care. *JAMA* 267(11):1511-1515.

Renaud, M. 1994. The future: Hygeia versus Panakeia?. In *Why are some people healthy and others not? The determinants of health of populations,* ed. R. G. Evans, M. L. Barer, and T. R. Marmor, 317-334. Hawthorne, USA: Aldine de Gruyter.

Rodney, P. A. 1997. Towards connectedness and trust: Nurses' enactment of their moral agency within an organizational context. Unpublished doctoral dissertation, University of British Columbia, Vancouver.

Royal Commission on New Reproductive Technologies. 1993. *Proceed with care: Final report of the Royal Commission on New Reproductive Technologies.* Canada: Minister of Government Services.

Roos, N. P. 1996. *Manitoba health care report.* Manitoba: Manitoba Centre for Health Policy and Evaluation.

Scanlon, C. 1996/1997. Impact of cost containment on patient welfare concerns nurses. *American Nurses Association Center for Ethics and Human Rights Communique* 5 (2):1-4.

Sherwin, S. 1992. *No longer patient: Feminist ethics and health care.* Philadelphia: Temple University Press.

Shindul-Rothschild, D. Berry, and E. Long-Middleton. 1996. Where have all the nurses gone? Final results of our patient care survey. *American Journal of Nursing* 96 (11):25-39.

Sibbald, B. 1997. Delegating away patient safety. *Canadian Nurse* 93 (2):22-26.

Starzomski, R. C. 1997. Resource allocation for solid organ transplantation: Toward public and health care provider dialogue. Unpublished doctoral dissertation, University of British Columbia, Vancouver.

Storch, J. L. and C. A. Meilicke. 1994. Political, social, and economic forces shaping the health care system. In *Nursing management in Canada,* ed. J. M. Hibberd and M. E. Kyle, 19-36. Toronto, Canada: W.B. Saunders Canada.

Thorne, S. E. 1993. *Negotiating health care: The social context of chronic illness.* Newbury Park, CA: Sage.

Veatch, R. 1991 Should basic care get priority? Doubts about rationing the Oregon way. *Kennedy Institute of Ethics Journal* 1(3):187-206.

Wachter, R. 1992. AIDS, activism, and the politics of health. *The New England Journal of Medicine* 326(7):128-133.

Walters, L. 1978. Ethics and the new reproductive technologies: An international review of committee statements. *Hastings Center Report* 17 (3):3-10.

Watson, S. D. 1994. Minority access and health reform: A civil right to health care. *Journal of Law, Medicine and Ethics* 22:127-137.

Wilson, R., L. Krefting, P. Sucliffe, and L. van Bussel. 1994 Native Canadians relocating for renal dialysis. *Can Fam Physician* 40:1934-1941.

Wolf, S. M. 1994. Health care reform and the future of physician ethics. *Hastings Center Report* 24 (2):28-41.

Chapter 14
Threats from the Western Biomedical Paradigm: Implications for Chinese Herbology and Traditional Thai Medicine

Edwin Hui, Sumana Tangkanasingh, and Harold Coward

In this chapter, two authors explore some of the threats to traditional and folk medicine posed by contemporary Western biomedical policy. Hui articulates these threats in terms of Canadian attempts to regulate Chinese herbology, while Tangkanasingh warns of the difficulties that traditional Thai medicine will have to transcend if it is to survive into the future. The former represents an effort by immigrant Chinese now living in Canada to retain some of their traditional values in the form of the employment of herbs for health maintenance and therapeutic purposes, whereas the latter may be seen as an attempt to preserve a rich tradition of medical practice which consists of strong religio-moral dimensions. Both reflect the intrusion of Western medicine based on the biomedical model into cultures and lifestyles which embrace vastly different values and worldviews with regard to human nature, health, and illness. Coward adds a concluding commentary.

Canadian attempts to regulate Chinese herbology

In Canada, all ingestible substances sold for human consumption, including herbs and botanical products, are classified either as foods or drugs and are regulated under the Food and Drugs Act and Regulations (FDAR).

Herbs as drugs

As drugs, herbal products generally fall into two major groups (Health Protection Branch 1990). The first group includes herbs listed in pharma-copoeias and major pharmacological reference works, with their properties, dosage, indications and contraindications for use well established. Products containing such herbal ingredients are reviewed in the same manner as other drug products and they are widely available on the market either as prescription drugs (e.g. digitalis, rauwolfia) or non-prescription drugs (e.g. lobelia, belladonna). The second group includes herbs which are not documented in the scientific literature but are traditionally known to be of medicinal use either on an empirical or anecdotal basis. The government considers that many of these references are useful in supporting the acceptability of herbal drug products, providing that the supporting references have not been superseded by more scientific research and study regarding toxicity (e.g. comfrey). In accepting herbal medicine in this second group, the government expects that they will be used for minor self-limiting conditions and prohibits any claims of their usefulness in the prevention or treatment of serious diseases, such as set out in Schedule A of the FDAR, or diseases which are otherwise inappropriate for self-diagnosis and treatment. These herbal medicinal products are to be designated as "Traditional Medicines" and must be labelled in such a way that the consumer should be able to judge the purpose of the product so as to use it appropriately. Furthermore, the government routinely reviews products intended for use in pregnancy, lactation, and childhood, or for use in circumstances where the ingredients might interfere with other medications or pose a hazard to persons with certain chronic physical disabilities.

In 1990, the Health Protection Branch published a mechanism for the registration of these herbal medicinal products as "Traditional Herbal Medicines" (THMs) (Health Protection Branch 1990). As part of the registration process, manufacturers must complete an application for each herb for a Drug Identification Number (DIN), and a proposed label must be submitted. In the application, each herbal ingredient must be identified, giving both its common and botanical name, and specifying the part of the plant used as well as the form in which the plant is present (e.g. powdered extract, tincture, etc.). The quantities of each of the herbal ingredients per dosage unit must also be provided. A clean claim or indication for the use of the THMs should be presented on the label, and their identities as medicines should be unequivocal in order to discourage a public attitude that they are foods or that they are innocuous just because of their herbal origin.

Herbs as foods

As foods, herbal products fall into these groups: (i) generally acceptable as foods; (ii) acceptable as foods under specified conditions; and (iii) unacceptable for use in or as foods.

A report (1993) prepared by an Expert Advisory Committee on Herbs and Botanical Preparation commissioned by the Health Protection Branch of the Ministry of Health list 74 herbs commonly sold in the market that have been reviewed and considered safe to be consumed as foods. The Committee also considered a second group of herbal preparations as acceptable as foods under specified conditions. This group of herbs may present a hazard under certain specific conditions, such as pregnancy, and are therefore required to provide cautionary labelling when sold as foods. A third group consists of a number of herbal substances which the Committee considered should be prohibited for use in or as foods and be added to the existing list of food adulterants in the Food and Drug Regulations. The following two criteria were used to determine whether a herbal substance is a food adulterant: (i) the potential of the substance for use as a food, including current or historical sale as a food product, and (ii) the margin of safety associated with the herb must be low or non-dose-related. The Committee generally agreed that toxicity should be the main concern in regulating herbs and recognized that long-term toxicity, as opposed to acute toxicity, is often the important concern in the consideration of herbal preparations. For example, it is recognized that comfrey has been widely consumed as a medicinal herb, a salad plant, and as a herbal infusion or tea. However, the symphytum species to which common comfrey belongs contain pyrrolizidine alkaloids that have been shown in animals studies to be hepatotoxic. This has been confirmed by reports of severe liver toxicity in humans consuming pyrrolizidine containing preparations. For this and other similar reasons, comfrey, along with 64 other plants, have been considered by the Committee to be adulterants when found in foods and are subject to control. Among the 64 herbs, twenty are Chinese herbs; and among the Chinese herbs, ten are used very frequently in traditional Chinese medicine. the list of herbs was published in Schedule 705 of the Canada Gazette (19 December 1992, Part 1).

Response from the Chinese community

The Chinese community was deeply concerned and responded quickly to these legislative initiatives, especially Schedule 705, demanding freedom of choice in the selection of health enhancing substances according to individual preference and cultural heritage. They were in agreement with the government as to the need to have reasonable control over toxic herbs and botanical preparations; where they differed was in their belief that some of the herbs listed in Schedule 705 should not be listed as adulterants and be controlled as such. They suggested that it is necessary to develop more culturally sensitive criteria with which herbs and botanical preparations may be classified and controlled. Moreover, it is crucial that people from all quarters involved in the herbal field (consumers, manufacturers, practitioners, and distributors) be represented in such an undertaking.

The Expert Advisory Committee named three new members in an attempt to comply with the request to increase regional representation. The newly formed Committee reconvened a meeting on 22–23 June 1993, and worked throughout the summer of 1993. The same Committee then presented its second report to the Health Protection Branch in October 1993, in which only five of the twenty Chinese herbs contained in Schedule 705 were reviewed; the remaining fifteen Chinese herbs are still undetermined, presumably regarded as drugs and controlled as such. In response, a local Committee for Preserving the Integrity of Chinese Herbology and Traditional Chinese Medicine was formed in 1994.

In the ensuing discussion between this Committee and the Health Protection Branch, many concerns have been expressed which have a cross-cultural dimension that deserves further consideration and comment.

To start with, the Chinese community felt that they were under-represented in the composition of the government Expert Advisory Committee. Among the ten members of that Committee, two are professors of Western pharmacology and of nutrition, two are business persons in Western herbs, one a retired professor, one a food industry consultant, two from the Canadian Association of Herbal Practitioners (all of the above are non-Asians); and one member of Chinese origin is an acupuncturist with training in Western medicine. Specifically, there is no expert of Chinese herbology and traditional Chinese medicine to speak on behalf of the Chinese herbal business communities and practitioners of traditional Chinese medicine. The Chinese community concluded that as a result, "the important values of time-honoured traditional Chinese medicine and Chinese herbs, the viewpoints of the Chinese herbal business communities, and the rightful position of traditional Chinese physicians may be totally ignored." (Committee for Preserving the Integrity of Chinese Herbology and Traditional Chinese Medicine 1994, 4) They strongly felt that this is unjustified in view of the fact that about 300,000 Chinese-Canadians reside in the Province of British Columbia alone.

In the second place, while members of the Chinese Committee agree that the toxicity of any herbal preparation has to be ascertained for the safety of the consumers, they feel that the way herbal toxicity is assessed betrays an insufficient understanding of Chinese herbology which has enjoyed a long history as one of the four pillars of traditional Chinese medicine.[1] The Committee indicates that in traditional Chinese medicine, the method of differentiating diagnosis and the principles of combining herbs to reinforce each other's therapeutic effects or to reduce and eliminate each other's toxic effects has not been taken into serious consideration. In Chinese herbology, herbs are applied in the clinical setting according to the combination of "king herbs", "subject herbs", "assistant herbs", and also on the basis of seven modes of relationships among herbs: mutual reinforcement among herbs, mutual assistance among herbs, fear and dislike among herbs, and so on. A given herb may be toxic by itself, but when it is used through herbal combinations commonly called formulas, which apply the different modes of herbal relationships, its toxicity is reduced or eliminated altogether. This is a unique feature of Chinese herbology which is fundamentally at odds with any known concept in Western pharmacology. Practitioners of Chinese herbology consider that any attempt to extract the chemical ingredient(s) from individual herbs for assessment of their toxicity demonstrates a lack of the understanding of the fundamental principles of traditional Chinese medicine and that following such a course would destroy the practice of traditional Chinese medicine in this country. Since Western pharmaceutical companies have extracted and identified active chemical ingredients from many Chinese herbs for the purpose of large scale chemical synthesis, such an approach would also be misinterpreted as government collaboration with the drug industry to unjustly exclude Chinese herbs from the market.

Similarly, a general lack of understanding of the theories and practices of traditional Chinese medicine can also be seen in the government's requirement to state the indications of these traditional herbal medicines in the terminology of Western medical symptomatology and therapy. For example, Section 2.6 (a) of the Directorate Guideline calls for a description of "specific symptoms likely to be relieved – e.g., 'expectorant, for the relief of productive cough', rather than 'for the relief of cold symptoms'." Also, Section 2.6 (b) requires that "claims and indications should be based on modern concepts of therapy. Terms such as 'tonic', 'supplement' … and other similar words are not acceptable". The community feels that greater sensitivity to and respect for the differences between the Western and Chinese medical systems should be shown in a multicultural society.

Finally, to facilitate the registration of herbs to be used as drugs, the Expert Advisory Committee of the Health Protection Branch has proposed to establish a series of "Standardized Drug Monographs" (SDM [herbal]). The purpose of these monographs is to facilitate the premarket review of products containing herbs. It is also recommended that the British Herbal Pharmacopoeia be used as a reference for the process of standardization. The Chinese herbal community considers the proposal to establish the drug monograph system impractical and unrealistic because of the large number of Chinese herbs involved. Also, the proposal to use the British Herbal Pharmacopoeia as a standard reference removes the use of herbal medicine from the context of the traditional Chinese medicine. The Chinese have at their disposal many established herbal pharmacopoeias compiled in the course of their long history, based on clinical experience and the theory of traditional Chinese medicine. Such time-honoured pharmacopoeias are clinically proven to be reliable and safe among the practitioners of traditional Chinese medicine and should logically be used to retain the integrity of the Chinese herbal system.

With the increasing appreciation and employment of alternative medicine, including herbal medicine, there is a great need to adopt an open-minded, honest, and sincere attitude to understand the values, beliefs, and traditions represented by these alternative medical systems. While the safety of con-sumers must be ensured, the manner to arrive at the standard of safety is the focus where sincere cross-cultural dialogue is needed.

The survival of traditional Thai medicine in the future?

Traditional Thai medicine is a product of local wisdom which is derived from long experience. We can classify traditional healers into four or five types: 1) traditional healers who use only medicinal herbs; 2) traditional healers who use both medicinal herbs and incantations; 3) traditional healers who use only incantations and mental power; 4) monk-healers; 5) masseurs. Unfortunately, traditional Thai medicine has survived only with some difficulty. After the coming of Western medicine to Thailand in the mid-nineteenth century, the teaching of traditional Thai medicine was given up officially in Thai medical schools (in 1923). After nearly a hundred years of receding popularity, traditional Thai medicine seems to be having its "renaissance" in the last decades of the twentieth century. Some even believe that traditional Thai medicine can be an alternative medical system in Thai society. The aim of this section of chapter 14 is to discuss whether Thai medicine can really be an alternative to meet current needs or if it is in fact a last choice in health care services.

As we come to the heart of the problem, we see a strong movement of romantic medical revivalism. During the last two decades efforts to promote traditional Thai medicine came from both government and private sectors, due in part to stimulation from the World Health Organisation. Mahidol University, for example, organized a seminar on "Traditional Medicine" at the Faculty of Medicine (1–3 October 1979) and suggested a policy to promote traditional Thai medicine for everyday life, to integrate traditional medicine with modern medicine, and to create organizations for these purposes. Two years later, Mahidol University and the Ministry of Public Health organized a seminar on "Medicinal Herbs and Primary Health Care" (11–13 February 1981) and presented findings on diseases which could be cured by herbs. Many research programs on medicinal herbs were subsidized. Thai massage was promoted in order to let people know how to relieve muscular pain by themselves. Even more impressive was the foundation of the Ayuravej Institute of Thai Traditional Medicine. This Institute was founded under the Ministry of Public Health, and an important conference on the "Thai Traditional Medicine Decade" was held 10–13 March 1995 at the Queen Sirikit Convention Centre in Bangkok. International co-operation contributed a great deal, especially in the case of a research program on the medicinal properties of five herbs (subsidized by Germany).

Moreover, various measures were proposed to develop traditional Thai medicine. These measures were, for example, to systematize the body of knowledge in traditional Thai medicine, to collect all data, past experiences, and writings in a well organized system, to examine the medicinal properties and toxicity of herbs, and to examine and improve the body of knowledge about traditional Thai medicine before selecting appropriate knowledge and techniques to be practised.

It is important to note that these measures represent the view of those who believe in modern biomedicine. But if the decision making comes from an authority which is totally Westernized, how can traditional Thai medicine be an equal alternative medical system? If we examine the regulation promulgated in 1967 by the Ministry of Public Health, one article implies a sense of superiority of Western biomedicine to traditional Thai medicine. "The practice of traditional healers means the healing practice which is derived from books or from training and that which is not scientific."

At the point of bringing together local wisdom and hi-tech medical science, there are limitations. We can see such limitations expressed in the speech of the ex-Minister of Public Health, Mr Chuan Leekphai (at Khonkaen Hotel, Khonkaen, on 23 March 1989):

> The data base on medicinal herbs is insufficient, scientific evidence supporting its use is incomplete, researches on this subject are too diversified, healers are unskilled and there is no assurance of safety.

This part of the speech of Mr Leekphai (who became the Prime Minister of Thailand between 1993 and 1995) may imply that the intention and efforts of those who have been trying to push forward traditional Thai medicine as an alternative medical system are an illusion.

However, is there another attitude toward traditional Thai medicine? In answer to this question we can examine other evidence for a clearer and a more vivid answer. Considering attitudes from many scholars in medical science, it seems that the biomedical and pharmaceutical conceptual frameworks toward medicinal herbs are the major factors. Such factors seem to be directing the Ministry of Public Health to take strict measures to control the use of medicinal herbs for the public – as if accumulated wisdom were not a subculture which has survived until now.

The main mistake of the effort to promote traditional Thai medicine is the promotion of this local wisdom out of its context and under the direction of Western medicine. Moreover, the distribution of medicinal herbs by district hospitals and small community health care units and the promotion of medical herbs without upgrading the healers manifest the negation of herbs as parts of traditional Thai medicine and the negation of the self-care system of the people. Besides, technocrats tend to forget that traditional Thai medicine does not mean only know-how in the use of medicinal herbs, but also includes the use of supernatural power.

It is believed by most traditional herbalists that medicinal properties not only exist in the herbs, but also come from a kind of supernatural power. This is the reason why some herbalists have secret rules in collecting herbs. For example, herbs must be picked on Tuesday; before picking, herbalists must ask for permission from Mother Earth; while picking it is forbidden to let the shadow of the herbalists lie on the plant. Moreover, during the mixing process (which in some cases is done by the patient himself), it is forbidden to talk, to let any person or any object pass over the boiling herbs, and when the preparation is over it is also forbidden for other persons to take that medicine. The efficiency of the supernatural power cannot, with our scientific instruments, be proved. But we cannot deny its psychological effects, as in the case of placebo. We can conclude that the efficacy of traditional medicine depends not only on the natural properties but also on the process of its preparation, the moral quality of the herbalist, the moral quality of the patient, the quality of the herbal distributor, and the social context (situation) of the distribution. Therefore, the distribution of traditional medicine in hospitals destroys the symbolic essence of the mystic sphere. Rooting out traditional medicine from its context is like getting rid of its curing power.

The current romantic medical revivalism in Thailand is not exempt from illusions and mistakes. The intent to substitute local herbs for Western medicine has not been successful. The efficacy of medicinal herbs has not yet been proven to be better than that of mainstream medicine. In cases of some small illnesses where traditional medicine can be used with good results, Western medicine is more popular because of its easier accessibility and its convenience. In contemporary Thai society, it is not only the lives of patients that have changed, but also the environment. Many of the forests have been destroyed, and in the same way main sources of medicinal plants have disappeared. Considering these factors, the substitution of imported Western medicine by traditional medicine is hard to realize in practice. The ideal of relying on ourselves, our own wisdom, and our own herbs, and the ideal of avoiding the side effects of mainstream medicine are accepted by well informed and well educated persons. However, these ideals cannot be reconciled with the need for efficient medicine for the whole nation at this point in time.

The future of traditional Thai medicine is not just an alternative medical service – an oversimplistic conclusion of a romantic planner. Nor can it be a last choice, because traditional Thai medicine is still a rich and mystic sphere to be discovered. Its contribution in the age of globalization is to give hope for patients who have tried modern medicine and failed. We should say that it gives us a last hope but not a last choice.

Conclusion

Both of the above case studies show how traditional medicine, in its interaction with the modern biomedical worldview, is in danger of being swallowed up. In the case of Chinese herbology, while the public policy approach of the federal government committee appeared to be sympathetic, in its judging of the potentially toxic herbs, it did so from the assumptions of how they would be used in a biomedical context. In doing so, the traditional knowledge of Chinese herbology was ignored, because of the different worldview and culture it represents. In cultural terms, one culture, the biomedical, is imperialistically judging the other, Chinese herbology, without having first made the effort to study and understand the quite different basic assumptions and long practical experience of traditional Chinese herbology. This is unethical at the policy level. Had true dialogue and understanding taken place, the federal policy committee would have learned from their Chinese counterparts that, although a given herb may be toxic by itself, when used in herbal combinations – the traditional "formulas" – the toxicity is reduced or eliminated. What is at issue is not just the availability of a particular herb, but the continuation in Canada of an ancient traditional medicine which is an integral part of Chinese culture. Canada's official embrace of multiculturalism policy needs to extend beyond food fairs and folk festivals to a real cross-cultural dialogue between traditional Chinese medicine in the form of herbology and modern biomedicine, which is the assumed culture embodied in federal committees and granting agencies. What the Canadian Chinese community requests is sufficient representation on federal committees of persons knowledgeable about Chinese herbology, so that a real dialogue between the two cultures can take place. Only then will an ethical rather than an imperialistic result be possible.

In the Thai example, the policy problem is parallel. Traditional Thai medicine is being placed under the control of the competing biomedical culture – ignoring the accumulated wisdom of traditional Thai medicine itself. Even the seemingly well intentioned government attempt to promote a revival of traditional medicine is shown to be fundamentally flawed because of being placed under the direction of authorities who are part of modern medicine and not knowledgeable about traditional medicine. The result has been a technological approach to the use of traditional herbs that ignores the Buddhist worldview within which the herbs have traditionally manifested their potency – the divine dimension is left out. Perhaps even worse is the crass economic motivation for using traditional medicine because it looks to cost less. In Thailand as in Canada, an effective co-operation at the level of applied medicine requires true dialogue between the cultures of which the competing medicines are but a part. Only when dialogue between the culture of modern biomedicine and the cultures of traditional medicines reaches a deeper level of understanding and mutual respect, will the formulation of truly ethical policy be possible. The prerequisite requirement for such dialogue is that modern biomedicine become self-conscious of its own assumptions, of itself as a culture, and stop imperialistically superimposing itself in committees and in government policy on traditional medicines and their cultures.

Note

1. The other three pillars are (i) acupuncture and moxibustion, (ii) massage and manipulation, (iii) dietary therapy and therapeutic exercises.

References

Canada Gazette, 19 December 1992. Part I.
Committee for Preserving the Integrity of Chinese Herbology and Traditional Chinese Medicine. 5 May 1994. *Statements.*
Health Protection Branch. 1990. *Drugs Directorate guidelines: Traditional herbal medicine.*
Health Protection Branch. 5 January 1990. Traditional herbal medicines. *Information Letter* 771.

Chapter 15
Global Challenges:
Ethical Implications of the Greening
of Modern Western Medicine[1]

Barry Glickman

The past two decades have *seen* a dramatic increase in interest in alternative health care options. This probably reflects both demographic and social factors. As the population ages, the inability of conventional Western medicine to deal effectively with chronic illness leads many to seek medical alternatives. Similarly, the human desire to delay the realities of aging stimulates interest in health promotion and food supplements. The cultural mosaic that is North America is also producing its impact. The millions of immigrants, particularly from the Orient, the South Pacific, and Africa, who continue to use their traditional forms of medicine, have greatly broadened our view of health care alternatives.

Today about 20 percent of North Americans opt for alternative health care treatments. While many prefer alternative health care because they are disillusioned with conventional medicine or have strong aversions to prescription drugs and surgery, the majority of alternative health care users hold the view that non-conventional approaches can supplement conventional approaches and use both simultaneously. There is also the perception that alternative health care approaches are less expensive than conventional medicine, though this will depend upon the health insurance regulations in the patient's home state or province.

Alternative health care options currently include chiropractic, acupuncture, therapeutic touch, homeopathy, herbal medicine, naturopathy, reflexology, and aromatherapy. Several of these approaches overlap in the dependence upon natural products, in particular homeopathy, herbal medicine, and naturopathy, though in the case of homeopathy, the treatments involve highly diluted preparations.

In addition to the formal use of alternative medical approaches, the public's interest in food supplements, food additives, vitamins, and minerals to maintain or improve individual health also depends upon the exploitation of natural products. This chapter examines the potential effect of the expanding market of natural products, primarily herbal, on the ecology of the planet and looks at the ethical aspects of eco-management. The driving forces behind the current interest in alternative medicine and health products are also considered.

Traditional healing and the greening of contemporary medicine

Traditional medicine is widespread throughout the world. Indeed, it is the common approach to health care for the vast majority of the world's population. It comprises practices that were in existence for many hundreds of years. It is defined by regional flora and fauna and by local religious customs and is therefore not directly transferable from culture to culture. In China, traditional medicine is an integral part of the health care system and is utilized in more than 40 percent of cases at the primary care level. Supplies are regulated through the state-owned Chinese Crude Drug Company. Formerly, crude drugs were collected in the wild, but as natural sources become depleted, many medicinal plants are cultivated in plantations that now exceed 330,000 hectare (Li Chaojin 1987).

The use of medicinal plants in North America occurs primarily in two forms. The first involves medicinal plants from which a single active ingredient provides the basis for a synthetic pharmaceutical product that can be patented. Motivation comes from the patent protection and prescription sales. The second involves crude drugs, and generally consists of dried plant parts or whole plant extracts. These can be sold in health food stores or as over the counter (OTC) remedies in pharmacies. They are thus used to treat self-diagnosed ailments, with or without a physician's advice. Examples of

OTC drugs include psyllium seed, cascara, sagrada bark, and senna leaves used in laxatives, or pseudo-ephedrine, an alkaloid from the *Ephedra* species (Foster 1995).

Green medications and food supplements in North America

"Green medications" are considered here to mean plant and/or animal products purported to have healing properties. These medications have generally not been subjected to scrupulous scientific testing, but often they have been used for hundreds, sometimes thousands, of years by humans for self-medication. "Natural products" in this chapter refers to the whole gamut of green medicines, herbs, dietary supplements (vitamins, minerals, and amino acids), and topical products which are available without a prescription.

Both North American concerns about health and diet and the fact that many non-conventional medications can often only be sold as dietary supplements shift the accent away from the use of traditional medications for treatment of common disorders, to more general health conditions. With our cupboards as full as they are, the question of whether we are feeding ourselves adequately, should never arise. Yet poor education, an unequal distribution of wealth, and the fast pace of our contemporary life-styles mean that many are not receiving adequate, let alone optimal, nourishment. Advertisements also continually inform us that our diet is so bereft of vital components that we need an extra boost of vitality through supplementation. This may indeed sometimes be the case, but to what extent are our new-found longevity, and stressful life-styles responsible? And, in whose interest is it to believe that we need supplements in the dosages that are sometimes recommended, and do we need as many of them as is suggested?

Perhaps the desire to heal oneself with natural products is part of the movement away from Cartesian thinking. Scientific materialism, which held that all things should be broken into their constituent parts to be examined scientifically, was also applied to the field of medicine. Modern Western medicine has followed this approach, and many feel the need for treatment in a more holistic manner – where the body is thought to be more than the sum of its parts. Because many suggestions in "health food" literature offer valid, wholesome alternatives to what has become the modern North American life-style, many readers also accept their suggestions of tenuous – even invalid – alternative medical treatments, many of which are espoused by prominent medical and athletic professionals. Consumers do not realize – nor are they meant to – the role of big business in manipulating the industry for commercial purposes.

There is a substantial profit (over $4 billion in the U.S. in 1993, according to *Fortune* 1995) being made in natural products, and consumers are being manipulated, sometimes lethally (*Cover Story*: "Drug Topics"). Disenchanted with conventional medicine and with the cost of medications, consumers often seek to cure themselves. And, in order to keep health care costs down and to avoid unpleasant confrontations, the authorities have been slow to act.

In North America, companies including Swiss Natural Sources, Essene Natura, Nature's Way, Quest, Natural Factors, and Life's Natural Wonders sell natural products, conjuring up images of Eden. Included among these products are food supplements, vitamins, and minerals. Nowhere is there a hint that most of the vitamins are synthesized in the laboratories of large chemical companies (Czap 1984). Proliferating on shelves of health food and drug stores, these products are promoted in legally acceptable ways to fill in the nutritional gaps created by what is commonly termed "our overly-processed diets". Natural products like vitamins, minerals, amino acids, and herbs fall under food or drug regulations in Canada's Food and Drug Act, depending upon their pharmacological activity.

Increased popularity and ecological pressures

A number of plants and animals of perceived medicinal value have been harvested to extinction and others are threatened with the same fate. An understanding of the environmental consequences of the expanding use of natural products requires consideration. In many cases controls prohibiting overexploitation are sorely needed. Unfortunately, the temptation for cash rewards often makes protection measures less than effective. Until recently, most of the interest in preserving species reflected fear of their loss through deforestation. The World Health Organisation of the United Nations has given credence to the estimate that 75–90 percent of the world's rural peoples rely on traditional herbal medicines and has called for a greater emphasis to be placed upon their use. They have also recognized that the greater exploitation of medical plants must be accompanied by conservation measures (World Commission on Environment and Development 1987). The International Union for Conservation of Nature and Natural Resources (IUCN) and the World Wide Fund for Nature (WWF) have developed plant conservation programs (Synge 1988) which includes an inventory and a data base. Co-operation with different countries has already led to the establishment of reserves for the protection of medicinal plants in Sri Lanka, Costa Rica, and Thailand. In some cases, these have also become centres for training, research, and development.

Does expanding popularity put plants and animals at risk?

Nature is by far our single most important source of medicines. The willow tree gave us aspirin, the belladonna plant produced the antispasmodic drug atropine, the chinchona tree gave us the antimalarial drug quinine, the foxglove plant gave us the heart medication digitalis. At least 50 percent of the prescriptions written in North America contain ingredients derived from nature, and over 25 percent of them include products extracted from plants. In some countries this fraction is considerably higher. In Germany, for example, more than 50 percent of prescriptions contain plant-derived ingredients.

The potential wealth of naturally derived medications is far from exhausted. Numerous natural products remain to be assessed for their medicinal value (Schultes 1986). As animals and plants become extinct, their possible contribution to human health is also forever lost. Those seeking a cure for hemophilia may never learn the details of the manatee's unique blood clotting properties, and if the rare desert pupfish disappears we may lose a cure for some kidney disorders.

The Pacific North West's yew tree (*Taxis brevifolia*) may serve to illustrate the importance of protecting natural resources. An extract of the yew tree, taxol, has been shown to have a positive effect on 30 percent of women suffering from ovarian cancer. Recently, the American cancer researchers requested protection for the yew tree as an endangered species. Old growth logging and prospecting for the tree have endangered its existence. About 60,000 pounds of dried bark will yield about 9 pounds of Taxol. It takes 2,000–4,000 trees to produce 1 kg of taxol, sufficient to treat 200–300 patients. As there annually are about 25,000 newly diagnosed cases of ovarian cancer in North America, about 500,000 trees would require harvesting each year. Don Minore at the Pacific Northwest Research station in Corvallis, Oregon, estimates the total stand of harvestable yew trees at only 1.2 million. Because of the demand, over 10,000,000 yew tree seedlings have been planted and alternative sources, including biosynthetic production, have been developed. The trees thus remain safe, though during the intense period of their exploitation in the wild, irreversible ecosystem damage was experienced locally.

Exploitation and diminishing return

Of 66 medicinal plants in use in Nepal, 47 are to be found in areas opened up by human activities. Of these, 5 are restricted to crop land, 11 to scrub forest, and 31 to other open habitats including trail sides and grazing clearings. In general, these plants have not been diminished due to current levels of human activities. The remaining 19 species appear restricted to shady, forested areas where the tree canopy remains relatively intact. One obvious conclusion is that deforestation would threaten these species. This is not an insignificant threat in communities where the need for firewood is greater than the regenerative capacity of the local forests.

Many Nepalese plants, however, have commercial value. The 12 most traded plants are 1) *Berberis asiatica,* 2) *Mahonia napulensis,* 3) *Lobelia pyramidalis,* 4) *Lyonia ovalifolia,* 5) *Swertia chirayita,* 6) *Cinnamomum tamala,* 7) *Rheum australe,* 8) *Rumex nepalensis,* 9) *Zanthoxylum armatum,* 10) *Valeriana jutamansii,* 11) *Acorus calamus,* and 12) *Paris polyphylla.* Of these, 4 are thought to have become less abundant in the past decade. The reduction in *Lobelia* and *Paris* may reflect deforestation while the scarcity of *Zanthoxylum* and *Valeriana* reflect over-exploitation. *Rauvolfia serpentina* (treatment of hypertension) and *Coptis teeta* (antipyretic) are over-exploited endangered species in India where an embargo on their export is in place.

Potential threat to medicinal plants

Many varieties of medicinal plants are threatened in America as well as throughout the world, and the push is on to cultivate these plants. As Foster says, "medicinal plant conservation ultimately means medicinal plant cultivation". Cultivation of lobelia not only increased its harvest, but also permitted selection that increased by 40 percent the concentration of its active ingredient, lobeline, which is used in over-the-counter (OTC) drugs to help smokers quit smoking. In 1994 the serious decline of eleven different herbs found mainly in the Himalayas caused India to propose restrictions on their harvest, and all eleven herbs are now being cultivated.

Unfortunately, cultivation does not often keep pace with harvesting from the wild, and popular species are disappearing. Because wild ginseng became so scarce in China, American ginseng was exported after its discovery in 1730, but the insatiable Chinese appetite for ginseng has created such a demand that now American species are threatened. Despite cultivation, 153,526 pounds of wild American ginseng was harvested in 1993, 95 percent of which was exported, mainly to Hong Kong. Wild American Echinacea, used as an immune-booster and antidote for snake bite and spider bite, is threatened because up to 100 tons are harvested each year. The Himalayan mayapple from which the anticancer drug podophyllum is semi-synthesized, is in serious decline.

Biodiversity, biotechnology, and medicinal plant conservation

Research into plants of ethnobotanical importance is also helping to increase our appreciation of plants. As an example, botanist Dr Nat Quansa and his students funded by a small grant from the World Wildlife Fund have catalogued more than 200 plants in Madagascar claimed to have medicinal properties. They include a creamy white orchid used to stop miscarriages, a fig that looks like a mango and is used to induce abortions, and an aloe that effectively stops infections. Other plants are claimed to relieve headaches, belly aches, tooth aches, diarrhea, and fever. Companies like Shaman Pharmaceuticals Inc. also help raise consciousness about the importance of plants by demonstrating interest in their potential commercial value.

Recognition of the potential loss of medicinal plants and genetic diversity has been a recognized consequence of the extensive destruction of plant-rich habitats, especially the tropical rain forests. The March 1988 conference in Thailand produced the Chiang Mai Declaration "Saving Lives by Saving Plants", which recognized the urgent need for international co-operation to protect and conserve natural resources. In addition, the Convention on International Trade in Endangered Species of Wild Fauna and Flora known as CITES was created to regulate trade in these species and their products. The effectiveness of these organizations, however, remains a matter of debate.

While plant species continue to disappear at an estimated rate of more than 400 species per year, the estimated value of a single plant species has been set at $203,000,000 (1985 U.S. dollars). Based on the estimation that 1 in 125 plants examined will have medicinal value, the estimated more than 2,000 plants that will become extinct in North America in the coming decade will have the staggering value of over three billion dollars. Although the argument that the commercial value of a species is an argument for conservation is distasteful, if not unethical, it has driven some countries to undertake a serious inventory of their plants. The Japanese government, for example, has dedicated a major facility in Tsukuba-shi to the cataloguing, collection, and seed preservation from plants around the world, their expressed goal being to have seeds from millions of plants available for scientific research whether the plant continues to exist in nature or not.

Data from NAPRALERT (Farnsworth and Soejarto 1991) indicate that about 9,200 of 33,000 species of plants or 28 percent of the plants on earth have been used ethnomedically. In China 14 percent of the plants have some drug application in that country. From this we can estimate that between 35,000 and 70,000 plant species have at one time in some culture been used for medical purposes.

Economic exploitation leads to commercial cultivation

With few exceptions, medicinal plants harvested in the wild can be cultivated. In India, for example, eleven medicinal plants, primarily from the Himalayas, were threatened with extinction by over-harvesting and were restricted in International Trade. Their economic potential resulted in successful commercial cultivation.

Trade in American ginseng (*Panax quinquefolius*) is monitored by the CITES. In 1993 the USA exported over 150,000 pounds of wild ginseng root ($141.80/lb). In the same year 1.5 million pounds of cultivated ginseng was exported to Asia ($36.43/lb). By way of contrast, only 6 pounds of wild ginseng was harvested in Northeast China, though a single root may fetch more than $10,000 in the Hong Kong marketplace. In British Columbia, ginseng has become a multi-million dollar agribusiness and questions about its impact on native land use and the extremely high use of pesticides in its production have become causes for concern.

Goldenseal (*Hydrastis Canadenis)* was introduced early as an anti-bacterial. It provided the alkaloids berberine and hydrastine which were until recently used in commercial eye care products. Most Goldenseal is harvested from the wild, mostly in the damp, beech forests of the northeast. It is still harvested in large quantities (150,000 pounds of roots per year) and sold primarily in health food stores and natural food markets. Current shortages are being experienced due to the over-harvesting of the wild plant roots. Goldenseal, however, can be cultivated and may soon become a commercial product produced under artificial shade.

One group of plants threatened by over-harvesting is the prairie species *Echinacea angustifolia. Echinacea* is used to treat infections. About 200,000 pounds of *Echinacea* is harvested annually from the wild. Farmers have successfully cultivated five species of *Echinacea.* Nevertheless, the harvest of wild plants continues unabated and regulatory steps will have to be taken to ensure the plant's survival in North America.

Evening primrose grows wild and along roadsides in eastern North America. Its edible roots and seeds are used for the treatment of atopic eczema and asthma. Indiscriminate harvesting, however, has put this species at risk and efforts to control its harvest have been initiated. Commercial cultivation of this plant should alleviate the pressure on the wild plant.

Saw palmetto (*Serenoa repens*) grows in the southeastern United States from the low coastal plains of South Carolina to the Mississippi and throughout Florida. The fruits of the palm are used in Europe to treat benign prostatic hyperplasia. Clinical trials indicate that it can be effective for this purpose. It is not yet under extensive pressure, and can be readily cultivated over large geographic areas which are of little use for other purposes.

The story of the rosy periwinkle: Setting the record straight

The exploitation of plants for medicinal uses is often associated with their destruction, at least in the popular mind. While it will be demonstrated that this can be the case, increasingly the recognition of the medicinal value of a plant is resulting in its cultivation and preservation. To illustrate with an example, contrary to the common belief (Strauss 1991), the curative benefits of the rosy periwinkle have not resulted in the destruction of the rain forests of Madagascar. In the first place, the rosy periwinkle is not a rain forest plant, but rather one that grows in open, drier areas. In the second place, for reasons of quality control, the plant is grown in greenhouses in Texas for pharmaceutical production, though it was once harvested by workers in

Madagascar as well as other places.

The rosy periwinkle is, however, a good example of a natural source of very effective medicines. The story of their discovery is also illustrative of how drugs are discovered from natural sources. In the early 1950s an American and a Canadian group were investigating the potential anti-diabetic properties of periwinkles in Jamaica and the Philippines. They did not find that the tea made from the plant leaves lowered blood sugar, but rather noticed a great reduction in white blood cell counts. This suggested that they might possibly be effective against leukemia. The Canadian group found one anti-cancer drug, vinblastine, while the American group found three, including vincristine. Vinblastine is highly effective against Hodgkin's disease while vincristine is effective against a certain childhood leukemia. Eventually two compounds were found that did reduce blood sugars, but these proved too toxic for human use.

Problems in protection

Among the many problems in international protection is the difference between the export of the plant versus its chemical product. An example is the genus *Podopyllum* or the mayapple which has a long historical use by native Americans. Mayapple's toxic root has been used to treat constipation, jaundice, hepatitis, fevers, and syphilis, and to induce vomiting, and expel worms. It was also used by Maine's Penobscot Indians to treat tumours and polyps. Today, derivatives of an active ingredient known as podophyllotoxin are used to treat testicular cancer and small cell lung cancer.

The Himalayan mayapple is the primary source of mayapple resin which is the primary source for the semisynthetic derivatives. Excessive decline in the wild mayapple population prompted India to propose that the mayapple be protected under the CITES treaty. The treaty does regulate the trade in the dried root, but not the chemical components derived from it. As a consequence, the protection process has done little to protect the plant.

The regulatory situation in Canada

Canada's Food and Drug Act has specific regulations regarding vitamins, minerals, and amino acids. Part D section 01.004 states that "no person shall, in advertising a food, or on a label of a food, make statement with respect to or any claim based on the vitamin content of that food". (*Food and Drug Act* 1978). According to the Canadian FDA, food is "anything you can swallow that isn't taken specifically for its pharmacological activity". It is thus illegal to state in advertising or on a label any benefits ascribed to the vitamin content of a food. This still leaves tremendous scope for spreading the gospel according to natural products – and this scope is extensively exploited. You simply have to read one of the surfeit of free health magazines available in any health food store. The point is that books, magazines, and pamphlets describing just how effective a given product is for a specific purpose in a descriptive fashion, not as an advertisement, are allowed!

Canada's health regulatory agency determines how a natural product is handled: "If it has identified distinct pharmacological activity, or claims on the label, it's a drug. If no claims are made and if it can be consumed without causing harm, it's a food." (Frank Welsh, Canadian FDA). This worked quite well until fifteen years ago, when there was a great expansion of "green" products on the market, including Chinese herbs, about which little was known. To regulate these products an expert advisory committee on herbs and botanicals was set up in 1985 by the Canadian government. In 1986, people from the health food industry and universities proposed a list of known toxic herbs to be considered as adulterants, and a list of some considered to be benign for all except pregnant women. In 1989 the resulting lists were published, then revised in 1992. Some five thousand letters and seven thousand signatures from consumers protested against these lists, forcing the advisory committee to reconvene to revise the lists again. Changes were made and the resulting report was published in February 1994 (see chapter 14 for more detail). Several products including Beetle Nut and Ginko Biloba are still under investigation.

Schedule 705 provides yet another revised list of herbs that will require informative labelling. The quality of natural products is set internationally by the World Health Organisation and the Sanitary and Phytosanitary agreement of the World Trade Organization. Nationally, standards are set by *Codex Alimentarius*, a joint program of the Food and Drug Agricultural department. Although other major countries such as Germany, Japan, France, England, and Australia allow health claims to be made on the labels of herbs, Canada and the U.S. will not. Herbs are considered as foods for which consumers can decide their use (Foster 1995).

To what degree should herbal medicines and vitamins be regulated?

Herein lies the conundrum: should natural products be allowed to make substantiated health claims if approved by a regulatory body, or should the situation remain as it is, with the product being offered for sale without any indication as to its possible beneficence? Should the consumer be protected by means of other legislation from the real possibility of harm caused by over-the-counter (OTC) natural products, or does the public have the right to decide what it wants? As the discussion of the previous chapter made clear, there are significant issues of cross-cultural ethics involved.

Should, for example, Chinese traditional medicines be regulated in the same way as prescription drugs? Should a standard level of training be required for the practitioners and dispensers? To make matters more difficult, not only have the treatments never been scrutinized by the same method of blinded clinical trials, the treatments are complex mixtures of plant and/or animal parts so that the quality of the materials is not uniform. Moreover, different communities will have different recipes and treatments for the same ailments.

It would seem reasonable that each of these communities be allowed to maintain their own traditions. The problem of course is that second and third generation patients are unlikely to limit themselves to a single form of treatment, but see both the traditional healer and the conventional physician simultaneously. Clearly the education of all parties involved is required. In time we can expect to see a *materia medica* (knowledge of the source, preparation, and application of drugs) of natural products made widely available to physicians so that potential negative interactions can be avoided. Great strides are being made in this direction with the increasing appearance of interactive CD-ROM publications containing such data.

Nevertheless, there is a need for some oversight. The lack of sufficient control over dietary supplements, coupled with health claims for natural products made by the health food industry, has had harmful, even tragic, consequences. Numerous examples have been reported (Muller 1982). Recently, β-carotene clinical trials were cancelled in several countries when increased, rather than diminished cancer rates were observed. It may, however, take years before these negative observations reach the consumer.

Dispute between vitamin proponents and the U.S. FDA

The war between vitamin proponents and the U.S. FDA dates back to 1962, when the FDA tried to establish more rigorous regulations for the sale and advertisement of vitamins. For the next ten years, the FDA participated in endless discussions and debates in defence against countless lawsuits. Responding to a 1972 recommendation by the Food and Drug Act to restrict labelling claims on labels of micronutrients and herbs, the U.S. National Health Federation (NHF), put together a well-orchestrated campaign to prevent this recommendation from being adopted (Herbert and Barrett 1985). The NHF appealed to congressmen and the general public. Former Congressman Craig Hosmer (R–California, NHF's headquarters) introduced a bill known as H.R. 643, which would have prevented the FDA from controlling vitamins. The NHF, which represents about 2,500 health food retailers, distributors, and producers, was giving free samples of health food products to congressmen between 1983 and 1985, and probably later. The NHF retains an attorney in Washington who files lawsuits and presents testimony repeatedly to regulatory agencies in order to minimize interference with the health food industry (Herbert and Barrett 1985).

Senator William Proxmire (D–Wisconsin) and Senator Richard Schweiker (who was later to become Secretary of Health and Services, the agency that oversees U.S. FDA activity) presented their own anti-FDA bill. In June 1973, *Consumer Reports* commented that Proxmire's bill would "reverse the trend of Federal law since 1938 requiring manufacturers to prove a product safe before it is marketed. It would require the FDA to prove a vitamin or mineral preparation unsafe before limiting its sale, an immensely difficult task" (Fried 1984). The bill passed.

In 1979, the FDA announced new proposals to treat vitamins and minerals as OTC drugs. Predictably, protest letters and phone calls besieged senators and congressmen. Senators Orrin Hatch (R–Utah, a state in which vitamins are an important industry) and S. I. Hayakawa (California) sponsored the "Voluntary Vitamin Act of 1981" (Fried 1984), which sought to remove FDA control over vitamins and minerals. The FDA backed off temporarily, then renewed its proposal to control supplements in the early 1990s. This time the FDA suggested that any claims as to the benefits of the contents of a product must be substantiated by scientific studies. The health food industry misinformed the American and Canadian public that this proposed legislation meant that consumers would not be able to buy vitamins and minerals over the counter.

Senator Orrin Hatch sponsored new legislation which would have required no "significant scientific" backing for health claims made on supplement labels (*N.Y. Times*, Oct. 1993). The campaign was successful, and in October 1994 Congress passed a law giving supplement manufacturers greater freedom in making claims about their products (*Fortune* 1995). William Jarvis, president of the National Council Against Health Fraud, decried the legislation, saying "The law is a disaster for the American public", because the onus was now on the FDA to prove that the dietary supplement was unsafe. Prescription drugs, however, must undergo rigorous testing to prove their safety before agency approval is gained. Even FDA nutrition scientist Lori Love bemoaned, "That is unlike all the rest of foods and all the rest of drugs and any other regulated product" (*Fortune* 1995).

Market influences

Domestic versus foreign markets

Supplements produced in Canada for Canadians must abide by Canada's regulations, while those made for export are not inspected or regulated, following only the guidelines set by the importing countries. Guidelines are often lax, and officials can often be easily bribed. Countries like Bangladesh, Mozambique, and Sri Lanka are successfully targeted, such that in

Bangladesh 25 percent of drug expenditures goes on vitamins (Muller 1982). Peter Schurch of La Roche, when asked his opinion regarding poor people who buy vitamins when what they obviously needed was food, replied, "Is it our problem? It can't be. We promote to the physician. The promotion reaches the public through the physician in nearly all cases I know" (Muller 1982).

Indeed, pharmaceutical companies do promote to the physician, beginning with medical school. Free black medical bags, summer jobs, and access to extensive medical and pharmaceutical literature, all contribute to the young physicians' comfort with the industry's presence. Ultimately, as practising physicians they will not only naturally prescribe the recommended products, but they have become dependent upon the companies for the easy access to presentable information (Lexchin 1984).

Use of medicinal plants and patent protection

According to Stephen Foster (1995), in his book *Forest Pharmacy: Medicinal plants in American forests,* investigation of plant medicines in the USA is extremely limited and there are essentially no studies describing how many plants could be harvested without threatening the wild population and its gene pool. Varro Tyler, Dean of the Schools of Pharmacy, Nursing, and Health Sciences at Purdue University, gives several reasons for pharmaceutical company reluctance to research American plants for their medicinal properties – difficulties obtaining patent protection. Because single chemical compounds are more easily assessed and patented, drug companies usually restrict research to these essences.

Expectations and realities

Humankind has always sought antidotes for disease from nature. Conventional medicine is, after all, the descendent of folklore and shamanistic cures. The promise of the scientific method as applied to medicine has not proven to be the panacea that many had hoped for, but perhaps we have been expecting too much. The amazing success of modern medicine may have fostered this very expectancy of delivery, and when it is not forthcoming, or is too expensive – when some still malinger and die from terrible afflictions – consumers become disenchanted and seek other cures. It is no wonder that articles informing us of the latest promising researches are so avidly embraced.

Ironically, pharmaceutical companies may temporarily stave off environmental destruction in their search for medicinal flora and fauna if they support indigenous research. For example, Merck & Co is backing a research institute in Costa Rica in their hunt for plants, micro-organisms, and insects with potential healing properties (Stevens 1992). For this endeavour, the government of Costa Rica is keeping 25 percent of its land untouched and will use some of Merck's funding for conservation. Another company in California, Shaman Pharmaceuticals, consults traditional healers in the Central Americas, and has a stake in the preservation of ecosystems.

Fads come and go, and harmful and useless products often fall out of favour. A nationwide survey of Americans released in 1990 by the National Association of Chain Drug Stores indicated that about 12 percent of former vitamin/mineral supplement users no longer took them. These respondents were most likely to be women, less than 40 years old, college graduates, and living in households with an annual income of over $35,000 (Gannon 1990). Thirty percent of them felt they "no longer needed vitamins", 15 percent thought they were too expensive, 15 percent said their diets were balanced enough, 11 percent believed that vitamins and minerals have "no effect on health" or "weren't helping" and 8 percent "felt ill when taking" supplements or "feel better without" them (*Cover Story*).

Extent to which pharmaceutical companies promote green medicines

The pharmaceutical industry has not raised any significant objection to the lack of regulation in green medicines because many pharmaceutical companies are in the field or have shown an interest in the green medicine market. Here are some examples:

The Swiss pharmaceutical company Sandoz established an affiliate in 1986 called "Sandoz Nutrition Ltd". Sandoz Nutrition has dived into the green medicine market with the acquisition of two of Europe's top health food brands, Eden and Dietisa. They have a presence in the natural food market through Céréal, Gerblé, and Reforma, and in pharmacies they sell the non-prescription supplements, "Milical" and "Minvitine". They also have a joint venture with the Italian company Gazzoni, selling the food supplement, "Lecinova".

Hoffman La Roche Ltd ("Roche") has a vitamins division, which supplies industrial clients worldwide with vitamins and carotenoids (Roche 1995 Annual Report). Roche has expanded this market with two joint ventures in China: It has a 70 percent interest in Roche Taishan to manufacture and sell vitamin A and has a 60 percent interest in Roche Sunve to sell Vitamin E.

Bristol-Myers Squibb has a consumer health affiliate called "Worldwide Consumer Medicines". The company's web site boasts, "The analgesics, skin care and other health care products of Worldwide Consumer Medicines compete in every major self-medication category".

The American pharmaceutical company Syntex formed a joint company in 1991 with the Hong Kong Institute of Biotechnology and the Chinese Academy of Sciences to screen compounds for their potential as pharmaceutical products and to discover the active ingredients of Chinese herbal remedies (*New Scientist* 1991). The large pharmaceutical company Pfizer Inc. has taken several steps into the green medicine market. In 1993, Pfizer purchased Charwell Pharmaceuticals Ltd, which distributes over-the-counter health care products. In 1994, the company paid $26 million for Restiva Italiana S.A., which sells health and skin care products. In the same year Pfizer acquired Rovifarma S.A., a Spanish producer of over-the-counter health products, for about $24 million.

In addition to active market involvement, the pharmaceutical industry has participated in discussions about natural medicines. In December 1994, the U.S. Food and Drug Administration (FDA) and the U.S. National Institute of Health's Office of Alternative Medicine jointly sponsored a symposium in Washington DC to discuss the use and regulation of traditional herbal medicines (Rowe 1994). The pharmaceutical industry participated in the symposium, which apparently raised more questions than it answered. A primary issue was whether the FDA could find less costly ways in which to grant approval of the low-technology medicines. Otherwise, only patentable products produce enough profit to justify the cost of complying with the FDA's stringent proof burdens.

Nature of the pharmaceutical industry's interest in green medicines

The pharmaceutical industry is interested in the green medicine market as a potential source of continued profit. As patents expire and competition increases, the pharmaceutical giants need new ways to make money. Mark Lange of Industrial Laboratories in Denver, states that pharmaceutical companies are aware of the increased demand for high quality nutritional supplements and that they are increasingly placing ethnobotanists on staff and establishing botanical supply lines.

The green medicine market is especially attractive in countries where their use is more accepted. For example, in Germany, 80 percent of physicians prescribe these medicines and they are covered by insurance (Rowe 1994). As of 1994, the German "Kommission E" put together scientific monographs of over 300 herbal medicines.

In general, however, the pharmaceutical industry's interest in green medicines is different from the existing green medicine industry. The pharmaceutical industry's primary goal is to use natural products to make patentable medicines.

The chief of the Natural Products branch of the National Cancer Institute stated that "no chemist can dream up the complex bioactive molecules produced by nature" (Raven 1995). Once such products are discovered, chemists can develop synthetic modifications. The synthetic modifications can then be patented, which translates to large profits. In 1988, natural products played a role in the top 20 pharmaceutical products sold in the U.S.

Given the prospect of profit, the pharmaceutical companies are taking a role in research and exploration of natural products.

Glaxo's web site points out that the ultimate goal of its plant research is to find a patentable medicine. The plants and soil are screened for activity against a specific biological target. The promising samples are then purified to find the specific substances responsible for the activity and are then examined further to find the chemical composition and molecular structure of the substance. The hope is that this will become a lead for the chemists to create a new patentable medicine.

Some say that the pharmaceutical industry's interest in green medicines is on the increase because of greatly improved drug-screening technologies and because of concern that the potential sources of medicines may disappear (Benowitz 1996). Norman Farnsworth, a pharmocognosist (one who studies the use of plants as therapeutics) at the University of Illinois at Chicago says that pharmaceutical companies are conducting more searches of the rainforest because of the "revolution in mass screening at a molecular level" (Benowitz 1996).

Reluctance of some pharmaceutical companies to sell green medicines

As seen above, the pharmaceutical industry certainly has the ability to enter and even take control of the green medicine market. Pharmaceutical companies can use their existing infrastructure to manufacture and market these products. The industry has plenty of cash to fund mergers and acquisitions as they have done in the health maintenance market and the biotech market. In 1995, the pharmaceutical industry spent about $4.5 billion in the financing of biotech firms (Holden 1996). Pfizer Inc. spent $115 million on four biotech companies in 1995. Glaxo bought the biotech firm Affymax for $533 million, and many other large pharmaceutical companies made similar acquisitions.

However, no such grand scale acquisitions have been reported in the green medicine market. Many pharmaceutical companies only devote a small portion of their drug research budget to plant based research (Benowitz 1996). Some companies believe that there is insufficient incentive to do research into the health benefits of natural products because of the lack of patentability and marketing exclusivity (Barnett 1996). DeFelice cited a published study, funded by Ocean Spray, that showed cranberry juice could be used to prevent urinary tract infections. All cranberry juice makers cashed in on the study, and because of the limitations of the U.S. Dietary Supplement Health and Education Act (1994), the only thing the companies could say was that their juice "promotes a healthy urinary tract" (Barnett 1996). The Quaker Oats company has been granted approval by the FDA to state "Eating oat bran or oatmeal daily may reduce heart disease risk"

(Brown 1996). However, bran is a non-patentable natural food substance, so any manufacturer can make the claim. In Canada, the Food and Drug Act and Regulations also prohibit health claims on foods or in advertising (*Food Focus* 1995).

David Trecker, head of central research at Pfizer, states that pharmaceutical companies will probably not take the lead in the green medicine market because of product and regulatory uncertainty (Brown 1996). He stated that the pharmaceutical industry has "so many diseases to attack directly with discrete drugs" and that "the economics [of patented pharmaceuticals] are so beneficial that to go with a murky natural product is a foreign concept". He says, "The thrust for this field definitely will come from the food industry".

James Miller (Missouri Botanical Gardens) states that some pharmaceutical companies are reluctant to sell green medicines because of the long, expensive extraction and purification process, combined with the fact that "ethnobotanicals" may only be effective by combining several ingredients, but the mixture of these ingredients is not patentable (Benowitz 1996).

Randall Johnson, director of bimolecular discoveries at SmithKline Beecham Pharmaceuticals in Pennsylvania states that, "pharmaceutical companies have been moving away from natural products with the advent of combinatorial chemistry" (Benowitz 1996). He stated that SmithKline no longer stockpiles thousands of plant, marine, and microbial extracts, which it once did.

Desirability of pharmaceutical companies selling green medicines.

There is a bit of a debate about whether pharmaceutical companies should enter the green medicine market. Herbalist Ranier Gertz of Edmonton accused the Canadian government of conspiring with the pharmaceutical industry when Ottawa proposed a list of 64 herbs to be classified as "adulterants" and subject to government scrutiny (Teel 1993). He stated that the pharmaceutical companies lose money when people get well through the use of herbs. Feather Jones of Turtle Island Herbs in Boulder is reluctant to see pharmaceutical companies enter the green medicine market because of the industry's poor harvesting and poor environmental record (Lange and Jones 1995).

Others would like to see green medicines sold as drugs, which presumably would invite the entry of the pharmaceutical companies into the market, provided there was marketing exclusivity. Barry Smith, as chief of the food regulatory branch of Health and Welfare Canada, has stated that the public must be protected from harmful natural products and products that are unacceptable for use in foods. He stated that if these products are used as drugs, they should be treated as drugs. The president of the Canadian Association of Herbal Practitioners agrees with Smith's view. Mark Lange of Industrial Labs welcomes the entry of pharmaceutical companies into the green medicine market, as he believes they will raise the herbal industry to higher standards.

Conclusions

Traditional medicine, including herbal remedies, can be an important supplement to conventional medical treatment. In several ways traditional approaches are better adapted to chronic illness and the maintenance of good health. While it is sometimes difficult to differentiate between the placebo effect and the actual medicinal value of treatments, alternative medicine also fills an important gap in the way Western society treats its patients. The time, personal attention, possible lower costs, and often the personal choice and personal involvement combine to make alternative forms of medicine attractive.

The popularity of alternative medicine also reflects the dissatisfaction of the user with conventional medicine. This in part may reflect the inability of conventional medicine to solve problems of chronic illness and the un-definable discomforts of aging. Western society has been characterized by its acceptance of neither an uncomfortable environment nor even fate, so there is no reason to expect members of that society to be content with its conventional medicinal practices. Moreover, as the society ages, the problems best treated by alternative methods will increase. Much of North America is a society with mixed traditions, spread out over an entire continent, and thus lacking strong family structures. With the baby boomers generally financially secure, rapidly loosing their parents, and aging them-selves, alternative medicine is appealing.

This fact has not gone unnoticed by the large commercial interests. One look at the shelves in any supermarket or drugstore will reveal that a trip to the health food store is no longer required to acquire alternative medications. What was once found on the shelves of the most "alternative" stores can now be found in the most conventional. The potential market is huge as judged by the size of the displays, the stacks of literature, pamphlets, and magazines as well as books on numerous health related topics. A quick scan of their contents reveals that they are essentially testimonials praising the products for health benefits that the laws of advertising do not permit.

At first sight, these retail outlets offer alternative medications for self-medication that do not require the extensive testing and assessment of prescription drugs. And, they must at some level compete with the conventional pharmaceutical products. Why then have they been tolerated by the influential pharmaceutical giants? It would be easy to force tighter regulation, more stringent quality control, and a strict limit on the supply of health claim information by the retailer. One potential answer is that the pharmaceutical manufacturers themselves play a major role in the production, distribution, and marketing of these products.

This raises a difficult ethical issue. The capitalist free-market principles permit the identification and creation of a market. Very little would be sold today if we were not first convinced that life without it would be impossible. Contemporary conditions are just ideal for the development of alternative medical treatments and health food supplementation. The first issue that then arises is the degree to which free-market policy should permit the exploitation of the consumer.

The second question which arises is whether there should be some epidemiological assessment of the value of these treatments, in particular of herbal medications. This would involve extensive funds whose source is not obvious. In addition, it would require quality control of products whose active ingredients remain mostly undefined – a difficult task, but some European countries, notably Germany, have developed some specified standards.

A third question of ethical consideration is the over-exploitation of the plants and animals used in traditional medications. Ample evidence indicates that both animals and plants can be harvested to extinction when the cultural or medical value of a rare product is sufficiently high. In North America too there is some past evidence that over-harvesting will occur. Indeed, as prices increase when the harvest is low, there is little disincentive to stop harvesting. One positive side effect of the commercialization of alternative treatments is that the commercial forces will tend to propagate the sales of materials that can be obtained and that sufficient infrastructure is thus available to assist in the cultivation of any commercially relevant species. Indeed, the overall, long-term threat of plant extinction within North America would appear to be quite small. The lack of regulations of the relatively low costs of overseas herbal markets may, however, not be so protective of the environment.

A final ethical question should ask who makes the decisions for the individual – the government, the conventional physician, the alternative health care provider, or the patient – and who should influence the decision making process.

Note

1. This report was made possible by the research assistance of Ms Mary McFadden and Mr R. Goldschmid LLB. Ms P. Tymchuk's assistance was invaluable in the preparation of the manuscript.

References

Adams, Stanley. 1984. *Roche versus Adams*. London, England: Jonathan Cape.

Alster, Norm. 1994. Natural partners. *Forbes* April:76.

Alster, Norm. 1995. Unseemly couplings. *The Economist* 13 May:66.

Astra. 1995. Annual Report.

Barnett, A. 1996. Neutraceuticals seek credibility in USA. *The Lancet* 347, 18 May:1397.

Benowitz, S. 1996. New technologies and approaches spur industry interest in plant derived drugs. *The Scientist* 10, 5 February (On-Line version).

Brown, K. 1996. Functional foods: A fruitful research field, but various regulatory obstacles persist. *The Scientist* 10, 4 March (On-Line Version).

Calgary Herald. 1987. Intake of minerals, vitamins often excessive, say experts. April :C1.

The Canadian Press, London. 1995. Herb sage may help beat Alzheimer's symptoms. *Times-Colonist* 19 Oct.:C1.

Cover Story. 1994. Drug topics. January.

Czap, Al. 1984. *Townsend letters for doctors*. Port Townsend, WA.

Drug Industry. 1984. Vancouver, Canada.

The Economist 1994. Heroic Doses. p.74.

Farnsworth, N. R. and D. D. Soejarto. 1991. Global importance of plants. In *Conservation of medical plants,* ed. Akerele et al.

Food Focus. 1995. Nutraceuticals: Functional foods an exploratory survey on Canada's potential. (June), Toronto, Ontario.

Fortune. March 1995:88.

Foster, Stephen. 1995. *Forest pharmacy: Medicinal plants in American forests*. North Carolina: Forest Historical Society.

Freundlich, N. 1990. Today's vitamin verdict: Take 'em, but not fistfuls. *Business Week*. 2 Dec.

Fried, John. 1984. *Vitamin politics*. Buffalo, NY: Prometheus Books.

Gannon, K. 1990. Americans don't often have facts about the vitamins they take. *Drug Topics*. 6 Aug.:24.

Glaxo Wellcome World Wide Web Site, http://www.glaxowellcome.com. Discovering modern medicines from natural products.

Herbal secrets. 1991. *New Scientist* 27 April.

Herbert, V. and S. Barrett. 1985. *Vitamins and "health" foods*. Philadelphia, PA: George F. Stickley Company.

Hoffman La Roche, Ltd. 1995. Annual Report.

Holden, C. 1996. Biotech on a roll. *Science* 271:151.

International Union for Conservation of Nature and Natural Resources (IUCN) Conservation Monitoring Centre. 1988. *Threatened primates of Africa. The ICUN red data book* ICUN Publication Services, Cambridge, UK

Lange, M. and F. Jones. 1995. When pharmaceutical companies manufacture herbal products: Two opinions. *Natural Foods Merchant* (On line version).

Lexchin, J. 1984. *The real pushers : A critical analysis of the Canadian drug industry*. Vancouver: New Star Books.

Li Chaojin. 1987. Management of traditional Chinese drugs. In *Role of traditional medicine in primary health care in China,* eds. Akerle *et al.*

Litwin, G. 1995. Jaws of life? *Times-Colonist*. 24 Oct.:C1.

Merck & Co., Inc. 1995. Annual Report

Muller, M. 1982. *The health of nations: A North–South investigation*. London.

Murphy, P. 1995. Fountain of youth banned by Ottawa. *Times-Colonist* 23 Oct.

Pfizer, Inc. 1995. Annual Report

Phalon, R. 1994. Dwayne's world. *Forbes* 154, 26 Sept.:20.

Raven, P. 1995. A time of catastrophic extinction. *The Futurist* Sept./Oct.:38.

Rosendahl, I. 1994. Surprising vitamin study stirs up controversy. *Drug Topics* 138, 5 Sept.: 39.

Rowe, P. M. 1994. Pharmaceutical populism at issue in USA. *The Lancet* 344, 24/31 Dec.: 1764.

Sandoz World Wide Web Site, http://www.sandoz.com, Sandoz Divisions: Nutrition.

Schultes, R. E. 1986 Ethnopharmacological conservation.: A key to progress in medicine. *Opera Botanica* 92:217-224.

Stevens, W. K. 1992. Shamans and scientists seek cures in plants. *New York Times* 28 Jan.: C8-9.

Strauss, S. 1991. Uncovering the truth behind the rape of Madagascar's rosy periwinkle. *Globe and Mail* 12 Sept.:D8.

Synge, H. 1988. *The joint IUCN-WWF Plants Conservation Program*. KEW:IUCN.

Teel, G. 1993. A prescription for herbs. *Alberta Report/Western Report* 20, 12 Apr.:50.

World Commission of Environment and Development. 1987. *Our common future*. Oxford University Press.

Part IV, Conclusion

Joan Anderson and Patricia Rodney

Listening to diverse voices

At the outset of Part IV, it was claimed that health policy must aim for public participation that is sufficiently diverse to represent a wide range of meanings. It was further claimed that achieving this would require critical self-reflection on the part of those who develop and implement health policy. Chapter 13 by Blue, Keyserlingk, Rodney, and Starzomski underscored the importance of both claims in a North American context.

Wolf (1994) warns that the professional–patient relationships most likely to flourish in our current North American era of cost containment will be those in which patients:

> [are] of a cultural background similar to the [professionals'], are not engaged in activities disapproved by the dominant culture and law, ... are not from population groups historically subject to bias within and outside the health care system, and ... have financial resources and a sense of options in their lives. (32)

In other words, at least risk are those who come from a culture that is congruent with the culture of the professionals who practise within the dominant biomedical paradigm. If public participation in health policy development and implementation is to make a difference here, we will need to become more critically self-reflective about what we mean by participation.

The concept of participation has become a key word in North American discourse on health, health care, and health research. Not only are we told that people should participate in decision making about their health and health care, but the notion of "consumer" participation extends to involving lay people in defining research problems in their community and in taking an active role in carrying out research projects. The pervasive ideology in some areas of research (such as health promotion research) is that people should have a say in what is researched, how it is researched, and how research findings are disseminated and used. This process, it is claimed, is in and of itself "empowering".

While we do not disagree with the intent of such participation, we feel that the ideology in which the intent is embedded obscures a number of issues. First, as was indicated in chapter 13, fundamental social inequities operate to exclude people from this participatory process. While participation is presented in ways that give the impression that the underclass in particular will now have a voice, in reality this is not the case. For instance, Anderson's research over the years has shown that a number of factors (particularly the contingencies of everyday life) operate in the lives of racialized women that exclude their voices from the discourse on health that takes place among middle class academicians and health care providers (Anderson 1996; Anderson et al. 1991; Anderson et al. 1997). Even if such women had the time or the inclination to participate in the discourse on health, the language of health professionals and the culture in which they operate exclude those who do not have access to the forms of thought and ways of speaking of the privileged. It is not just lack of English language skills that exclude people; even those who speak English might find no common ground of understanding with middle class health professionals and academics.

But there is a further point that needs to be recognized. Women, such as those who speak in Anderson's research, are active agents who have their own notions about health and the health practices that they wish to use in their families. They may look to the professional sector for illness care and the notion of participation may have little meaning to them. Health may be viewed as encompassing domains of spiritual well-being, domains that might be best managed in the family through holistic healing practices that are far removed from Western "health care/illness care" systems. Such alternate views of health were certainly portrayed by Hui and Tangkanasingh in chapter 14 and by the authors in Part III. Participating in programs to promote health that deal with health in a mechanistic way (e.g. diet and exercise) may be of little interest to those who conceptualize health as encompassing a more holistic perspective on life.

The issue then is that the very notion of participation as conceptualized within our current North American discourse is constructed from within a eurocentric cultural perspective of health and illness. People who do not share this eurocentric belief system may not expect to participate in decisions regarding medical care or health care as constructed by Western middle class professionals and by government bureaucracies – even in such locations as Thailand (as chapter 14 shows).

In terms of participation in research, the very notion of research may be seen as having no relevance to the everyday lives of people who are consumed with making a living on a daily basis. Research as we know it might well be of interest only to privileged academics, professionals, and major industries such as pharmaceutical companies. Furthermore, a very real danger of participatory research as we see it emerging in the North American context is that what might be presented as working with a community may in fact be an appropriation of knowledge in the guise of participation. Of late, since the rhetoric of participation has gained momentum, participatory research has become fashionable. What this seems to mean is that researchers are out looking for people from "ethnic communities" to be on their research teams; the danger is that communities might derive no benefit from the research, and might find themselves simply supporting academics and health professionals in their research in a manner no different than the more traditional approaches. It could be argued that the kind of participatory action research advocated by people like Paulo Freire (1970) in his *Pedagogy of the Oppressed* bears little resemblance to the popular version that has evolved among North American academics and politicians. The context was different and so was the motive.

This is not meant as an indictment of public participation in decision making about their health or in naming the research that ought to be done in their communities. Far from it – we have argued in chapter 13 that public participation is urgently required in both North America and Thailand. Our point is that there is danger in employing any policy concept or program of action without reflection. We need to be more thoughtful about the issues that are germane to public participation and recognize that the popularizing of this process may be to the detriment of the individuals and communities who most need to have a say in their health care. Moreover, we need to recognize that communities are not homogeneous entities with common interests; intra-group divisiveness and relations of power are usually the reality within any given community. We will have to take up these challenges if we are to listen effectively to diverse voices in the development and implementation of health policy.

Opening spaces for multiple views

It was also claimed at the outset of Part IV that health policy must not limit its attention to dominant Western biomedical views of health and health care delivery. In chapter 14, Hui illustrated the tensions that arise when Western biomedicine collides with traditional medicine. And Tangkanasingh illustrated that such tensions arise transnationally. In other words, when countries import Western biomedicine, they also import elements of the culture within which it is embedded, a culture that does not easily make room for other ways of approaching health and health care.

Opening spaces for other ways of viewing health and health care will require more critical scrutiny of the power of the Western biomedical paradigm. To a large extent, that paradigm is dominated by military and market metaphors (Annas 1995). These metaphors emphasize "the quest for control that seems to define both modern medicine and postmodern politics" (Annas: 747). And, as Glickman demonstrated in chapter 15, too often the consequence is an appropriation and commercial exploitation of traditional and folk culture. Indeed, critics have warned that such appropriation and commercial exploitation is an extension of Western colonization (Shiva 1997).

Towards global health policy

In concluding, we wish to return to our comments in the Introduction about the social determinants of health. Health is not necessarily equated with health care; it has a great deal to do with how a society looks after economics, employment, education, crime, and so forth (Renaud 1994). This was a point that was supported by Blue, Keyserlingk, Rodney, and Starzomski (chapter 13) in their discussion of inequities in North America. Other empirical work also emphasizes the importance of the social determinants of health. For example, in exploring the environment and health in Central and Eastern Europe, Hertzman (1994) depicts how political and economic stresses are linked to environmental degradation and serious health consequences.

Improving the health of populations in North America, Thailand, or anywhere else requires dealing with the social determinants of health – determinants that are affected by an increasingly global economy (Laxer 1996; Shiva 1997). Thus, in bringing to a close our cross-cultural dialogue on health policy, we wish to call for a reconceptualization of social justice.

This reconceptualization should address the circumstances of peoples' lives and their differing worldviews, not just the distribution of health care services. This reconceptualization of social justice must make room for global economic and political analyses if we are to improve those circumstances.

References

Anderson, J. M. 1996. Empowering patients: Issues and strategies. *Social Science and Medicine* 43 (5):697-705.

Anderson, J. M., Blue, C. and Lau, A. 1991. Women's perspectives on chronic illness: Ethnicity, ideology and restructuring of life. *Social Science and Medicine* 33 (2):101-113.

Anderson, J. M., Dyck, I., and Lynam, J. 1997. Health care professionals and women speaking: Constraints in everyday life and the management of chronic illness. *Health* 1(1):57-80.

Annas, G. J. 1995. Reframing the debate on health care reform by replacing our metaphors. *New England Journal of Medicine* 332 (11):744-747.

Freire, P. 1970. *Pedagogy of the oppressed.* (M. B. Ramos, Trans.). New York: Continuum.

Hertzman, C. 1994. Environment and health in Central and Eastern Europe: A report for the Environmental Action Programme for Central and Eastern Europe. Washington: The World Bank.

Laxer, J. 1996. *In search of a new left: Canadian politics after the neoconservative assault.* Toronto: Viking.

Renaud, M. 1994. The future: Hygeia versus Panakeia?. In *Why are some people healthy and others not? The determinants of health of populations,* ed. R. G. Evans, M. L. Barer, and T. R. Marmor, 317-334. Hawthorne, USA: Aldine de Gruyter.

Shiva, V. 1997. *Biopiracy: The plunder of nature and knowledge.* Toronto, Canada: Between the Lines.

Wolf, S. M. 1994. Health care reform and the future of physician ethics. *Hastings Center Report* 24 (2):28-41.

Chapter 16
Conclusion

Robert Florida

When we started this project some five years ago, none of us really knew how challenging it would be. Perhaps if we had, we might not have volunteered so readily. As scholars we often found it hard to operate at the level of cross-cultural sensitivity and intercultural dialogue that we call for in health care ethics. Our different academic disciplines, national and cultural backgrounds – not to mention temperaments – were barriers that we constantly tried to negotiate in order to understand the issues and to come up with some relevant cross-cultural insights and perhaps even some solutions to practical problems. Did we succeed?

I believe that we did come to the point where individuals in the group actually did begin to see issues in new ways, ways that had been learned through cross-cultural insights. Some of this comes through very clearly in the book. For example, the suggestion that some sort of notion of interdependence or "we-self" should challenge the dominance of the singular autonomous "I" as the centre of value in modern Western biomedicine comes from our consideration of Thai Buddhist, Hutterian, First Nations,

Chinese, and other viewpoints.

This idea has obvious applications in day-to-day clinical work in the multicultural Canadian context, but even at that level it is not always easy to apply. The Chinese and First Nations practice of families having the duty to take decisions about individual members' health care does not fit very well in practice with how Canadian hospitals deal with the problem of informed consent. Similarly the Chinese filial responsibility to conceal the knowledge of a terminal condition from parents conflicts with the biomedical ethical approach to informed consent and to the related issue of the patient's right or responsibility to know the full nature of his or her condition.

In Parts III and IV there is also evidence that this cross-cultural venture was fruitful. The chapters in those sections, which build on the preceding theoretical discussions and expositions of individual cultural views, show the authors to have benefited from the cross-pollination that came from working with such a diverse group of participants. These chapters are perhaps the most original contributions of the book and could hardly have been written by scholars working in isolation. Our central themes of the study – that Western biomedicine is an imperialistic culture in itself and that social determinants of health are of primary importance even though too often shunted aside in health care ethical discourse – are not particularly cross-cultural insights. Nonetheless, bringing them into the analytical foreground is a valuable contribution of this study.

On the issue of effecting fundamental changes to the direction that biomedicine is taking around the globe, our study finds little reason for optimism. In the discussions of the status of traditional medicine in Thailand, of Chinese herbalism in Canada, and of corporate exploitation of "green" medicine, it is all too clear that biomedicine has very successfully taken the dominant position. The ancient naturalistic traditions must struggle to find a niche where they can be tolerated and allowed to survive. On the level of respecting First Nations' cultural values, the K'aila story suggests that biomedical technical views will simply sweep aside spiritual considerations.

Similarly, we note that the issues concerning the social determinants of health, more honestly "ill health", in Canada's First Nations discussed in this book have not changed significantly for many decades and still seem of very little interest to our provincial and federal policy makers. In Canada, Thailand, and other countries today there is considerable public interest in health care policy issues. It is our hope that the insights and concerns found in this study will not be forgotten in the debates that continue. We believe that our cross-cultural approach shows the danger that would follow from uncritically continuing along the biomedical path which demands the technological domination of nature for the benefit of the individual while ignoring the interconnection of each of us to family, society, and nature.

About the Authors

Joan M. Anderson is Professor of Nursing at the University of British Columbia School of Nursing. She received her PhD in sociology from the University of British Columbia in 1981. She works primarily in the area of culture and health, anti-racism in health care, and women and health. She is the author of a number of articles on various aspects of health care, culture, and women's health.

Arthur W. Blue is a Professor Emeritus at Brandon University, a retired clinical psychologist, a former psychological advisor to Health Canada, and psychological consultant to Corrections Canada. He was the first president of the Native Psychological Association in Canada, the Society for the Advancement of Native Studies, and Chairman of the editorial board for *The Canadian Journal of Native Studies*. He has been involved with a number of international research projects including: Child of Two Soils, International grant to study the cross-over effect in North American Indian children, Tiyospaye Project, NIMH grant to study the effects of traditionality on health on the Rosebud Reservation. Alzheimer's Study of North American Indians, NIH grant to examine the incidence of Alzheimer's in Indian communities. He is the author of a number of articles dealing with mental health and acculturative stress in Aboriginal peoples of North America.

Michael M. Burgess is a philosopher, specializing in bioethics. He currently holds a research chair in Biomedical Ethics at the University of British Columbia's Centre for Applied Ethics, the department of Medical Genetics, and a clinical appointment to the B.C. Children's Hospital. Following completion of his PhD at the University of Tennessee, he was on the Faculty of Medicine at the University of Calgary, and served as an ethics consultant to hospitals and a regional health care unit. His current research utilizes qualitative research methods to assess the effects of genetic technology on family relations and on society, specifically in the areas of Huntington disease and breast cancer. Other recent work is in cross-cultural health care ethics.

Harold Coward is Director of the Centre for Studies in Religion and Society and Professor of History at the University of Victoria. His main fields are comparative religion; psychology of religion; and environmental ethics. He serves as an Executive Member of the Board, Canadian Global Change Program. His wide variety of publications include *Pluralism: Challenge to World Religions* (1985), *Population, Consumption and the Environment: Religious and Secular Responses* (SUNY Press, 1995), and *Life After Death in World Religions* (Orbis, 1997).

Robert E. Florida is Professor of Religious Studies and Dean of Arts at Brandon University. His current research interests are in Buddhist ethics and health care ethics. He has recently served on the board of the Canadian Bioethics Society and has organized bioethics workshops for the community in Brandon, Manitoba.

Barry W. Glickman is a Professor in Biology and Director of the Centre for Environmental Health at the University of Victoria. He received his PhD in Molecular Genetics from the University of Leiden in 1972 and works primarily on the relationship between the environment and cancer with a particular interest in the origins of mutation. His research has included studies on the genetic effects of radiation, including both accident victims and Soviet cosmonauts, and the role of DNA repair in determining individual predisposition to cancer. He is an editor of *Mutation Research* and on the editorial board of *Environmental and Molecular Mutagenesis*.

Barry Hoffmaster is a Professor in the Departments of Philosophy and Family Medicine at the University of Western Ontario. From 1991 to 1996 he was the Director of the Westminster Institute for Ethics and Human Values in London, Ontario. He served as President of the Canadian Bioethics Society in 1994-95, and he has been a Fellow of The Hastings

Center since 1995. He is a co-author of *Ethical Issues in Family Medicine* (Oxford University Press, 1986) and a co-editor of two collections of essays and one text in bioethics and one collection of essays in journalism ethics.

Edwin Hui is Associate Professor of Medical Ethics and Spiritual Theology and Associate Dean in charge of the Chinese Studies Program in Regent College, University of British Columbia, where he received his MD and PhD and theological training. He is a Research Associate of UBC's Centre for Applied Ethics and Ethicist of the B.C. Cancer Agency and since 1995 Visiting Professor to the Department of Philosophy and Religion of Peking University. He is the founding editor of the *Regent Chinese Journal*, and his research interests include the interface between medicine and theology, and religion and culture. His recent publications include two edited volumes in ethics entitled *Questions of Right and Wrong* (1993) and *Christian Character, Virtues and Bioethics* (1996), and a volume in religious studies entitled *Dialogue: Confucianism, Buddhism, Daoism and Christianity* (1997).

Edward Keyserlingk is Associate Professor in the Department of Social Studies of Medicine and Director of the Biomedical Ethics Unit, Faculty of Medicine, McGill University. He is also Director of the Ethics and Law Teaching Program in the Faculty of Medicine and Clinical Ethicist at the Montreal General Hospital. He did his graduate studies in both ethics and law and received his PhD from McGill University in 1983. He works in both bioethics and health law with a particular interest in cross-cultural perspectives in both disciplines. Among the publications authored is *Sanctity of Life and Quality of Life in the Context of Medicine, Ethics and Law* (1979). He is presently editing a book on cross-cultural aspects of the interaction of ethics and law in biomedicine.

Michael McDonald occupies the Maurice Young Chair in Applied Ethics and is the founding Director of the Centre for Applied Ethics at the University of British Columbia. He is the author of various publications in applied ethics, including *The Ethics Reading Handbook* (for the Certified General Accountants of Canada) and *Towards a Canadian Research Strategy for Applied Ethics* (for the Social Sciences and Humanities Research Council of Canada). He has also published in ethics, political philosophy and philosophy of law, especially in the area of minority collective rights. McDonald served as Deputy Chair of the Tri-Council Working Group on Ethics that produced The Code of Ethical Conduct for Research Involving Humans. McDonald is past-President of the Canadian Philosophical Association and the former Editor of *Dialogue*.

Pinit Ratanakul received his PhD in Philosophy from Yale university and is the Director of the Center of Religious Studies, Mahidol University, Thailand.

Sheryl Reimer Kirkham, RN, MSN, is a Doctoral Candidate at the University of British Columbia, School of Nursing. Her dissertation research is a critical ethnography of "Intergroup Dynamics in Health Care Provision in a Pluralistic Society", with a focus on processes of racialization. This research builds on her Masters Thesis "Nurses' Descriptions of Caring for Culturally Diverse Clients". She was formerly on faculty at Camosun College, Victoria, as Nurse Educator and has published and presented on topics such as cross-cultural nursing, research methodology, and nursing curriculum.

Patricia (Paddy) Rodney is an Assistant Professor at the University of Victoria School of Nursing in British Columbia (Lower Mainland Campus). She is also a Research Associate with the University of British Columbia (UBC) Centre for Applied Ethics and Providence Health Care Ethics Services. Dr Rodney teaches and consults in health care ethics, and is a member of the ethics committees of B.C. Women's Hospital, St Paul's Hospital, and the North Shore Health Region.

Dr Rodney graduated from the UBC School of Nursing's PhD Program in the spring of 1997. Her studies have included an extensive focus on health care ethics and feminist ethics. More specifically, her feminist ethnographic research focuses on how nurses deal with ethical problems in their practice, and on how the culture of the health care system impairs the moral agency of nurses and other members of the health care team.

Peter H. Stephenson is Professor of Anthropology as well as a faculty member in the Centre for Environmental Health at the University of Victoria. He received his PhD from the University of Toronto in 1978. He has also served as editor of the journal *Culture* and as president of the Canadian Anthropology Society. He is author of *The Hutterian People* and senior editor of *A Persistent Spirit: Towards understanding Aboriginal Health in British Columbia*. He has also written many journal articles and book chapters. Professor Stephenson was the 1997 recipient of the Weaver-Tremblay award given by the Canadian Anthropology society for achievements in applied anthropology. He has worked with many immigrant and refugee communities in Canada, with First Nations communities, and in the Netherlands, on issues related to health care, aging, and the environment.

Rosalie Starzomski, RN, PhD, is Assistant Professor at the University of

Victoria School of Nursing in British Columbia (Lower Mainland Campus) and a Research Associate with the University of British Columbia (UBC) Centre for Applied Ethics. She is an Ethics Consultant at the Vancouver General Hospital, a member of the Vancouver General Hospital Ethics Committee, and is involved in teaching and consulting in the area of health care ethics and health policy. Dr Starzomski received her PhD in Nursing from UBC in 1997 and her dissertation "Resource Allocation for Solid Organ Transplantation: Toward Public and Health Care Provider Dialogue" examined moral reasoning around ethical issues related to organ transplantation as well as community participation in health care decision making. Her current research is focused in the areas of health care ethics, health policy, organ transplantation, nephrology, and genetic testing.

Khannika Suwonnakote, RN, PhD, is a graduate nurse faculty member of Ramathibodi School of Nursing, Mahidol University ,Bangkok, Thailand. She is a former Vice Dean in Nursing Affairs, Faculty of Medicine, Ramathibodi Hospital, Mahidol University, former director of the Graduate Program in Nursing. She also is a chair of nursing ethics development committee and a chair of the Nursing Ethics Course of the undergraduate nursing curriculum.

Sumana Tangkanasingh received her Doctorat du troisième cycle in sociology from Grenoble University and is teaching in the Department of Humanities, Faculty of Social Sciences and Humanities, Mahidol University, Thailand.

Subject Index

Aboriginal culture 1, 5-8, 10, 54, 149, 151, 158, 162-8, 176-87
abortion 1, 125, 133
advance directives 183, 190-6, 216
aging 19-81, 84, 87-8, 236
AIDS 26, 29-31, 107, 147, 202
"alternative" medicine 103, 236-254
anthropology 50, 52, 69, 79-80, 83, 130, 177
antibiotics 82-3
antibiotic resistant bacteria 70, 82-3
Asia 1, 6, 104
autonomy (see also identity) 7, 10, 123, 131, 140-4, 148, 150-2, 158, 162, 165, 176, 182-7, 191-9, 203-4
balance 37-42, 55, 59, 201
bioethics (see also health care ethics, medical ethics) 1, 72-4, 76, 106, 139-40, 157, 160-1, 164, 167-8, 174, 192-5, 204

biomedical paradigm 10, 56, 227-231, 233, 258
biomedicine 24-5, 34, 43, 50, 56, 58, 60, 69-70, 79, 93-9, 103, 157, 169-70, 176, 203, 213, 226, 231-2, 264
biomedicine as culture 3, 5, 10, 63, 69-71, 80, 113-4, 159, 264
biomedicine–traditional medicine relationship 1-11, 34-5, 44-5, 104, 176-87, 203-5, 213, 226-35, 236-54, 260, 264
Boorse 9, 95-105, 114
Buddhism 2, 4, 6-10, 17-33, 41, 119-26, 133, 168-70, 201-4
Canada 4, 10, 54, 56, 61, 75-7, 104, 117, 150, 170, 173, 218-20, 227-31, 234-5, 244-6, 264
cancer 9, 20, 29, 48, 77, 85, 107, 147, 240-1, 244, 246
care givers 187, 190-2, 194, 197, 199-